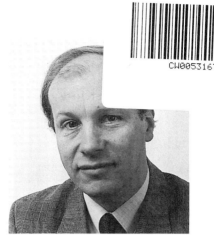

John Cochrane MS, FRCS is Consultant Surgeon at the Whittington Hospital, London. His interest in teaching started before he began to study medicine when he spent a year teaching in a school in Jamaica. He has been Undergraduate Sub-dean at the University College and Middlesex School of Medicine and is now Postgraduate Dean and Director of the Academic Centre at the Whittington.

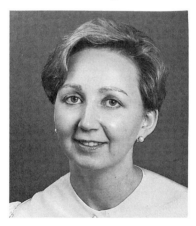

Anne Szarewski DRCOG, trained initially at the Middlesex Hospital Medical School, London and then in Obstetrics and Gynaecology at the Royal Northern and Whittington Hospitals. She currently works as a Family Planning Doctor at a Well Woman clinic, as a clinical assistant in genito-urinary medicine at St Thomas's Hospital, London, and as a clinical assistant in colposcopy at the Royal Northern.

THE BREAST BOOK

John Cochrane MS, FRCS and Dr Anne Szarewski

Recommended by the Family Planning Association

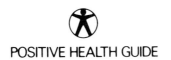

POSITIVE HEALTH GUIDE

© John Cochrane and Anne Szarewski 1989

First published in 1989 by
Macdonald Optima, a division of
Macdonald & Co. (Publishers) Ltd

A member of Maxwell Pergamon Publishing Corporation plc

British Library Cataloguing in Publication Data

Cochrane, John
    The breast book.
    1. Women. Breasts. Diseases
    I. Title   II. Szarewski, Anne   III. Series
    618.1,0089

    ISBN 0-356-15416-5

Macdonald & Co. (Publishers) Ltd
66–73 Shoe Lane
London EC4P 4AB

Photoset in 11/12pt Times by
🅰 Tek Art Ltd, Croydon, Surrey

Printed and bound in Great Britain at the
University Press, Cambridge

CONTENTS

ACKNOWLEDGEMENTS

We would like to thank our families for their patience and endurance during the writing of this book.

We would also like to thank all at the Highgate Group Practice for their many valuable suggestions, and also our editor, Harriet Griffey, for her continuing encouragement and support.

The publishers would like to thank Maggie Raynor for her line illustrations; Wyeth Laboratories for the breast self-examination photographs; the Middlesex Hospital for the photograph of breast dimpling; BUPA for the mammography photograph; Dorling Kindersley Limited for permission to use their illustrations from *Everywoman's Medical Handbook*; Nancy Durrell McKenna for the mastectomy photographs; and Spencer (Banbury) Limited for the photographs of prostheses. Cover photograph by the Robert Harding Picture Library.

INTRODUCTION

Most women worry about their breasts at some time or other in their lives. They may be anxious about the appearance of their breasts, about premenstrual heaviness, tenderness, or a lump – the range of problems is wide. It is such an important topic that there is now information available from a wide variety of sources. There are leaflets about breast screening, articles in newspapers, television documentaries, not to mention friends with information that may be confusing, contradictory and sometimes actually incorrect.

This book seeks to provide a comprehensive up-to-date guide; most of the information is not available from any other single source. We have attempted to set out the facts as completely, as clearly and as honestly as possible. We have included medical terms because we believe that women need to talk the same language as the doctors they consult. Doctors in the past have tended to disguise their knowledge (or lack of it) by using complicated long-winded words. The terms used here are all explained and are not difficult to get to grips with.

Women need this information because there is so much they can do to help themselves, and so much they can do to prevent problems arising in the first place. In addition, many of the decisions that have to be made about breast problems have no clearcut medical basis and depend to a large extent on the woman's views. What may be the right decision for one woman will not be best for another. A woman therefore needs to be involved in any decisions about her breast problems. However, she cannot be involved unless she has access to the facts. Questions like 'Do you want tablets for your breast tenderness?', 'Do you want your benign lump removed?', 'Will you agree to be entered into this trial?', or 'Do you want plastic surgery for your breasts?' are difficult to answer, particularly if all the information she has is the little that the doctor can put across in a brief consultation. Often the reply is 'Well I'll leave it up to you doctor, you know best.' It used to be thought best that doctors decided how to manage childbirth, which they considered as just another 'disease', but now it is accepted that the mother should make decisions about this natural process.

Fortunately most of the breast problems that do arise are minor and quite harmless, but any thoughts about breast problems are dominated by anxiety about cancer and the operation of mastectomy. This happens because breast cancer is the commonest of women's cancers, affecting one woman in 14. It might be that awareness of this fact, along with all the other details about breast cancer given in this book, would produce even more anxiety, but generally the unknown is more worrying than the reality. It is better to know that 90 per cent of breast lumps are harmless, that even cancer can be successfully treated, and that new, safe and satisfactory alternatives to mastectomy are now available than to worry in ignorance.

So this book covers the whole story of breasts, from childhood to old age. We hope that the information it contains will be a positive promoter of good health, and that, rather than raising any anxieties, it will bring the confidence that you can get by having a better understanding of yourself and your body.

1

THE STRUCTURE AND FUNCTION OF THE BREAST

INTRODUCTION

The shape of the female breast, together with its function of producing milk, combine to make it the essence of femininity. It fulfils its maternal role perfectly, allowing the baby to nestle in the mother's arms at a comfortable distance for visual contact while it takes in an ideally-mixed liquid diet through the conveniently-shaped nipple. The baby can hear the comforting sounds of the maternal heartbeat transmitted directly to the ear through the breast.

In fact all mammals have breasts, but the human breast has an additional component, an infilling between the milk-producing cells, that gives the breast this softness and its characteristic shape. This texture makes the breast soft and comforting for the baby, and its rounded shape gives the breast its sexual appeal.

STRUCTURE OF THE BREAST

The breast lies partly on the ribs, which can make feeling for lumps more difficult, and partly on the pectoralis muscle. The pectoralis is a large fan-shaped muscle covering the chest, and it has a small effect on the size of the breast, depending on how well developed it is. The breast has an 'axillary tail' that stretches up into the armpit (axilla) and can sometimes be mistaken for a lump. Looked at from the side, the breast often has a slightly concave contour above the nipple and a convex one below it.

1

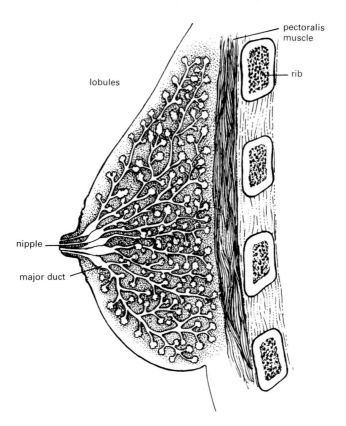

Cross-section of the breast.

Milk is produced by specialised cells in the lobules of the breast, from where it passes through small ducts to the 15 or so major ducts which open separately onto the surface of the nipple. These major ducts act as reservoirs of milk. The lobules are surrounded by fat and this two-component structure of the breast often gives it a naturally 'lumpy' feel. The weight of the breast is supported by fibrous suspensory ligaments that run through the breast substance up to the skin, and which tend to stretch with age. They can also give warning signals of malignant disease deep in the breast by pulling in or 'dimpling' the skin.

The nipple is surrounded by the areola, a disc of muscle, at the edge of which is a ring of sebaceous glands that produce an oily secretion. During lactation this secretion helps lubricate and protect the nipple from the rigours of suckling. The skin over the areola is sensitive and when it senses that the baby is starting to suck it stimulates the areola muscle to contract and this pushes the nipple out to make sucking easier. This same sensitivity also makes caressing the breasts and nipples a part of sexual arousal.

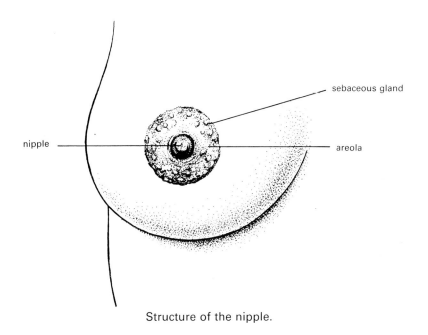

nipple

sebaceous gland

areola

Structure of the nipple.

Lymphatics
Blood flows to and from the breast through the arteries and veins, but there is another circulation system. This transports a straw-coloured tissue fluid called lymph in a separate set of channels called lymphatics. Most of the lymphatics from the breast run towards the axilla (the armpit), where they pass through filters called lymph nodes. If the lymph contains any germs such as bacteria the nodes filter them out, sometimes getting enlarged and tender in the process, just as nodes in the neck sometimes get enlarged after a sore throat. Similarly, if a malignant cell from a lump has got into the lymph channels it may be filtered out in these axillary lymph nodes and either be destroyed there or perhaps make them enlarge.

3

DEVELOPMENT OF THE BREASTS

Before birth

Breast development begins in the embryo at about the sixth week, following patterns laid down in our distant mammalian past. Two ridges of nodules appear along the front of the embryo, mimicking the rows of nipples in other mammals. These gradually disappear, leaving just two, high on the chest wall, which later develop into the breasts. Occasionally one or both of those breast buds disappear too, leading to the congenital absence of the breast, a condition for which there is no treatment, apart from cosmetic surgery. Less rarely, some of the extra or accessory nipples are left behind, but it is extremely unusual for these to cause any trouble.

Birth

At birth, babies of both sexes often have quite distinct breast nodules, as a result of the mother's high levels of breast-stimulating hormones acting on the baby's breast tissue. Occasionally these nodules secrete a whitish fluid, known as 'witch's milk' in the past. Once out of the womb and away from the mother's hormonal influence, the nodules fade away, and breasts remain quiescent until the beginnings of the adolescent surge in endocrine (hormone) activity.

Puberty

During childhood, boys' and girls' breasts are identical. However, during puberty very profound changes take place in girls' breasts, due to the interaction of the pituitary gland (the conductor of the endocrine orchestra) with the ovaries.

In girls the ovaries start secreting a hormone called oestrogen, which stimulates the tiny ducts in the breast to elongate and to branch. It also causes the changes in the areola and the nipple which become obvious a long time before the first period occurs. Sometimes the rapid enlargement of the breasts causes temporary stretch marks in the skin.

The other ovarian hormone, progesterone, is necessary for the growth of the milk-secreting glands at the end of the ducts, although these do not actually produce milk until they are influenced by the hormones of pregnancy and lactation. Much to their embarrassment, adolescent boys can also develop breast nodules during this time of hormonal turmoil; however, they disappear in time, and should be left firmly alone.

4

The age of onset of puberty in girls (the menarche) is very variable. In exceptional circumstances puberty can occur in early childhood, but it needs investigation in case there is some underlying problem or disease. At the other end of the scale, a girl who has not started her periods by the age of 18 should also be investigated. General health and nutritional state play a large part in determining the age of puberty. As a country becomes more affluent and girls are better fed, the age of menarche falls. In early nineteenth-century England, for example, the average age was about 17; now it is 12½.

Various things can go wrong during the development of the breasts. Occasionally they just don't seem to know when to stop, and the girl is left with enormous, heavy and uncomfortable breasts, that are not only unsightly but can cause a lot of embarrassment and interfere with social and sporting activities. Surgical breast reduction, however, leaves unsightly scars and makes breastfeeding in the future impossible. Alternatively, the breasts may fail to develop adequately. This can be dealt with more easily, either by hormones or by surgical breast augmentation. Both these operations are described in Chapter 8 on cosmetic surgery. Sometimes the breasts are unequal in size, or the nipples are particularly large, bifid (with a cleft in the middle) or hairy. These problems are rarely serious, but may cause considerable embarrassment. The influence of advertising or the media sometimes makes women unhappy about the development of their breasts. Often all that is needed is a discussion with your general practitioner to get these worries and concerns into perspective.

Maturity

During adulthood the breasts are greatly influenced by fluctuations in the levels of the ovarian hormones, which change throughout the monthly menstrual cycle. Most women notice alterations in the size, heaviness and sensitivity of their breasts during the month, and occasionally this can result in uncomfortable tenderness that is bad enough to warrant treatment. The increase in size of the breasts that may occur before a period is due to accumulation of fluid within the breast tissue.

During sexual arousal the muscle of the areola contracts when stimulated, so that the nipple becomes erect, and a flush may extend over the front of the chest.

Pregnancy

The next great change comes with pregnancy. High levels of the hormones oestrogen and progesterone, with the assistance of other hormones called prolactin and human placental lactogen, stimulate the secretory glands of the breast, elongate the duct and increase the fat deposits, making the breasts generally bigger, all in preparation for lactation (milk production).

Breastfeeding

After the baby has been born a hormone called oxytocin is produced by the pituitary gland which stimulates the tiny muscles in the ducts to contract and squeeze the milk towards the nipple. Thereafter, putting the baby to the breast causes these muscles to contract in a reflex fashion – the so-called 'let-down reflex'. The force of these tiny muscles will be familiar to anyone who has witnessed the way milk squirts out of the nipple during breastfeeding.

Once breastfeeding is established, there is a close relationship between the amount of milk taken by the baby and that produced by the mother, making a very economical link between supply and demand. As the baby is weaned, less milk is taken, so less is produced, and the supply gradually falls but sometimes stopping breastfeeding leads to very tender engorgement of the breast.

Menopause

At the menopause, when the ovarian hormones fail, the glandular tissue in the breast shrinks, to be replaced usually by fat. The fibrous supports stretch, so the breasts tend to drop, unless supported by a good bra. At last the breasts are released from the hormonal see-saw, and so hormonally induced conditions such as tenderness at some point during the menstrual cycle (cyclical mastalgia), cysts and certain lumps (fibroadenomas) cease to be a problem.

2

MAKING SURE YOUR BREASTS ARE ALL RIGHT

If a problem is going to arise in your breasts, then it is only sensible to find it at the earliest stage, when it can be treated by the simplest and most effective means. You can help yourself to do this in four ways:
- Examining your breasts regularly.
- Finding out how breast problems start and what to look for.
- Attending a screening session if you are in the right age group.
- Not delaying seeking help if you have a possible breast problem.

SELF-EXAMINATION

Most women today have a fair idea of the techniques of breast self-examination, and have heard of the recommendation that they should examine their breasts every month. However very few women do this regularly – probably less than one woman in 10. Many feel guilty and anxious because they know they 'ought' to, but they still cannot bring themselves to do it.

Reluctance about self-examination
The reasons why self-examination is neglected are very understandable. The first problem is that normal breast tissue is lumpy anyway, and feeling for lumps may just create anxiety. Also, when you have never felt a breast cancer, it is very difficult to go feeling for one in your own breast. Many women say they are 'squeamish' about feeling their breasts. Some are worried they might damage such soft delicate tissue

7

by squeezing it. And many women are just too busy and forget, or do not have the opportunity in terms of a warm room, an appropriate mirror and freedom from interruption for self-examination.

Perhaps more important than any of these often-given reasons is that to examine oneself is to accept the unthinkable – that there might actually be a cancer there. 'There's nothing wrong with me. I feel well. Why should I look for trouble?' For this reason the examination is often done hurriedly and superficially.

Does it matter if it is not done?

Some women prefer to make occasional, perhaps yearly, visits to a breast-screening clinic or to their doctor instead. However a woman doing a self-examination every month is going to get to know her own breasts very well; so well in fact that, even though she does not have the medical experience that a doctor has, she should still be able to detect lumps earlier than they would be found by occasional visits to a doctor. She is much better able to remember where her normal lumpy areas are and to notice any changes.

Even though regular self-examination is rarely carried out, most breast lumps are still found by women themselves. They are discovered when washing in a bath or shower, rubbing suntan oil into the skin on holiday, or rubbing oneself after a knock. Sometimes they are noticed by a partner or friend. It is much less common for them to be found for the first time by a doctor or at a screening clinic. The two unfortunate consequences of this are, first, that the finding of lumps comes as a much greater shock because of the worrying uncertainty about how long the lump has been there, and, second, lumps are often larger than they would have been if regular checks had been made.

It could be argued that if more self-examinations were done there would be more false alarms and more anxiety created. In practice it seems that the more regularly it is done the greater is the knowledge about what is normal for you, and the fewer healthy 'lumpy' areas are interpreted as unhealthy lumps. Furthermore, the major advantage is that a true lump will be found at an earlier and, if it turns out to be malignant, at a more curable stage.

One sad aspect of looking for breast lumps is that many

8

women, mostly in the older age group, find lumps and then tell no-one about them. Partly there is the hope that, until a doctor actually says it is a cancer, it might not be a dangerous lump. However there is also the fear of going through all the treatment that may be needed and of the general upset this will cause. And sometimes the woman has little doubt that the lump really is a cancer but attributes it to some previous bump or bruise.

TECHNIQUE OF SELF-EXAMINATION

When it should be done

The examination does not need to be carried out more often than once a month, and it is best to do it just after the period has finished because there will be less breast tenderness and less lumpiness then. If you are no longer having periods then the start of each calendar month is the easiest time to remember.

It needs to be done preferably in a warm bedroom or bathroom and without interruptions. Although it should not be rushed, it takes very little time.

Looking at your breasts

Start by undressing to the waist and sitting or standing in front of a mirror in a warm room. Face the mirror first and then turn from side to side. Look for differences between the two breasts. These might be:
• Differences in size
• Differences in nipple height

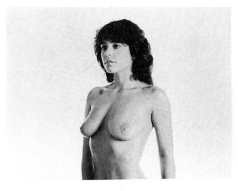

Then look at each breast separately for:
• Irregularity in its normal smooth contour
• Any dimpling of the skin
• Any drawing in or retraction of the nipple
• Changes in the texture of skin such as puffiness
• Changes in the colour of the skin
Do this with your arms down at your sides to start with, then with your hands on your waist, then with your arms stretched out above your head and finally with your arms behind your head.

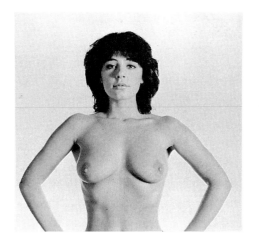 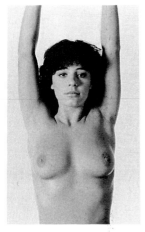

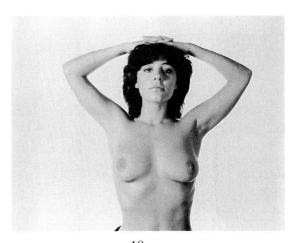

Of course there will be some differences between the two sides. An important reason for doing a visual examination regularly is that you will get to know what is normal for you and be able to look for changes.

Feeling your breasts

Next lie down on a bed or in the bath. Before you start feeling the breast it is important that the breast tissue is evenly spread over the chest wall so that there are no folds that you might mistake for lumps. You can do this by rolling slightly away from the side to be examined and putting the arm behind your head.

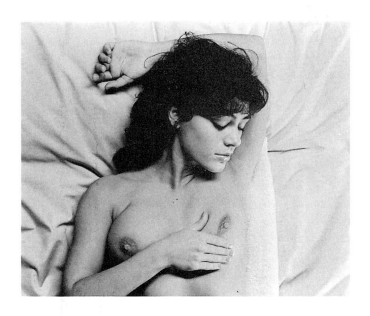

Examine the right breast with the left hand and vice versa. It is most important to feel the breast with the flat part of the middle three fingers and to work systematically round the breast. Develop a routine if you can – work your way gradually around the breast, moving your fingers in small circles so that you check each area. When you have finished that, repeat with the other breast.

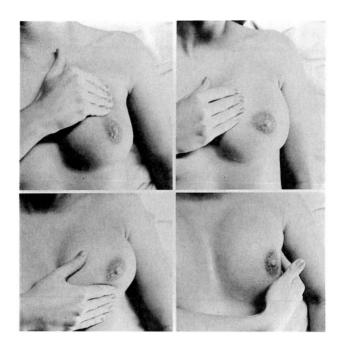

It is easy to feel false lumps with the fingertips or by pinching, but what you are looking for is:
- A lump that can be felt with the flats of the fingers.
- A lump that moves up and down and from side to side with the breast tissue (so it is not a rib).
- A lump that you can tell fairly clearly where it starts and stops (what is called a discrete lump, that is clearly distinguishable from the surrounding tissue).

Any abnormal lump that you find is likely to be about the size of a pea or larger. Lumps the size of a grain of rice are almost certainly not significant. If you are not sure whether there is a lump in one area, for instance in the axillary tail of the breast, where it is often 'lumpy', compare it with the same area in the other breast. It is not important to be feeling for tender areas, just for lumps.

Also as part of a regular check you should look at your clothes for any nipple discharge – although there is no need to squeeze your nipples to see if you can produce a discharge.

12

Lymph nodes

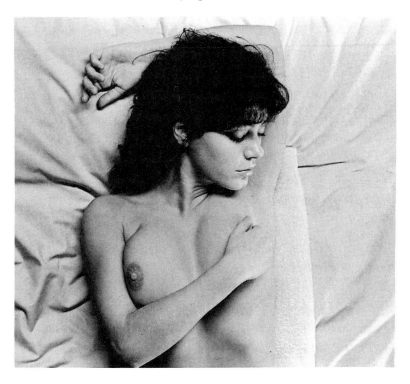

Finally feel in your armpit for lymph nodes. If you are examining your left breast have your left arm down by your side. Get your right hand up as high as you can into your left armpit and then slide it down over your ribs. It is often possible to feel normal nodes (you can often feel normal ones in the neck and groin as well). Again you are looking for changes; an abnormal one is likely to be bigger than the size of a pea.

How would a cancer show itself?

A breast cancer is usually discovered because it produces a lump in the breast. The lump usually feels irregular and its texture is firmer than that of the surrounding breast. It is also usually discrete, meaning it is possible to feel where the lump starts and stops. It may be the size of a pea or larger when found, in any part of the breast and either quite close to the

13

skin or deep down in the breast. It is rarely tender – pain from it is unusual.

Even when quite small, a cancer may produce a change in the outline of the breast or dimpling of the skin as it pulls on the suspensory ligaments of the breast. Sometimes these changes on the surface are the first signs that there is a cancer within the breast, and this is an important sign to look for.

Very occasionally the first sign of a breast cancer is a watery or blood-stained discharge from the nipple. Alternatively there might be a change in the skin of the breast – either a change of colour or the skin getting puffy or firmer. The finding of an enlarged lymph node producing a lump in the armpit is another way that a breast cancer can be discovered.

Even without ever having felt a cancer before, these signs are usually fairly easy to detect. Of course some breasts are more lumpy than others and then it can be difficult, even for the most experienced of specialists. However the cause of delay in discovering a cancer is usually due to the woman not looking, rather than by any difficulty in recognising what is found on examination.

And it is important to realise that even if you find all these 'characteristic' signs of breast cancer, they can just as easily be caused by simple benign conditions. Of course, it is understandable to jump to the conclusion that a lump must be cancer, especially if it has some of the characteristics mentioned above, but unless the diagnosis has been proved by a biopsy then there are plenty of other possibilities (as you will find in Chapter 5).

SCREENING CLINICS

Better than looking for cancers when they have got large enough to feel is to find them at the earlier (and more curable) stage when they are too small to feel. That is the aim of breast screening.

Breast-screening clinics have existed for many years, and are often called well-woman clinics. They may be set up by the local health authority, either in the community in health centres or in family planning clinics, or within hospitals. Some are privately run and some are run by large firms for their own employees; for instance in 1976 Marks & Spencer set up a mammogram-based screening programme for all their female staff over the age of 35. Women may go to most of these clinics either if they have breast problems or for a breast-check even with no symptoms, although each clinic will have different criteria as to who they will screen.

Starting from 1988, the Department of Health and Social Security has been setting up a comprehensive range of screening clinics throughout the country, in response to the Forrest Report published in 1987. Invitations to attend are being sent to all women aged between 50 and 64 – a total of 4,857,500 women – on behalf of their general practitioners. The screening will involve no examination but just a single-view mammogram, and the mammograms will then be repeated every three years.

MAMMOGRAPHY

Mammography has emerged as the most satisfactory way of finding breast cancers before they produce a lump that can be felt. Other methods such as thermograms (measuring the heat produced by different areas of the breast) were tried in the past but they were less satisfactory. Ultrasound is a good way of looking for breast cancers in women under the age of 35 for whom mammograms are not helpful (because the breast tissue is too dense), but it is less suited to screening large numbers of patients.

A mammogram is simply an X-ray taken with a special machine designed to show up the internal structure of the breast, and is simple and quick to do (Chapter 5 describes what happens when you go to have a mammogram). In the past it has always been standard practice to take two X-ray pictures of each breast, one taken from above and one taken from the side. The new screening clinics carry out a single oblique, i.e. 45-degree, view on each breast. This is a simpler and quicker technique, although the pictures are more difficult to interpret. Fortunately most breast cancers have a particular characteristic that makes them show up on these special X-rays; they get little spots of microcalcification in them, due to calcium being laid down in the blood vessels of the tumour, and these appear as tiny white dots on the X-ray. There are often signs of thickened tissue pulling on the suspensory ligaments as well.

Not all breast cancers have these white spots of calcium, or at least in some patients changes in the rest of the breast may mask them, but mammography is still a very good screening technique. There is evidence from a study in New York that cancers may be found on average two years before they would have been otherwise detected, while a Swedish study showed that mammography will pick up 86 per cent of those cancers otherwise expected to arise in the following year, and a large proportion of those cancers that would not otherwise show themselves until even later. Studies in Holland reported in 1984 suggested that women are only about half as likely to die of breast cancer if they were regularly screened by mammography, and a Swedish study showed a 30 per cent reduction in mortality from breast cancer, although the benefit was confined to those women over 50. In some of these studies an examination was carried out as well, and how much extra benefit this gives is difficult to decide.

What is clear, however, is that if examination discovers a lump in the breast, a mammogram is not going to help in the treatment of that lump. A subsequent biopsy will almost certainly be needed, whatever the mammogram shows, although sometimes a mammogram is still needed to look at the rest of the breast.

Problems that might arise with mammograms
Sometimes there is a need for a further X-ray to be taken, and this is always a particular cause for worry for the woman. It happens especially if only a single oblique view has been carried out. After a single-view screening it is estimated that about 10 per cent of women will be recalled for a conventional two-view mammogram; these further pictures will show that seven out of ten of these women do not have cancer and the other three will need further tests. This has led some people to suggest that it might be better if two-view mammograms were used for screening; however, even single-view mammograms on 4.8 million women every three years is such a major undertaking that it is the only practical way to start such a programme. This question will need to be kept under careful review, though.

Often the changes found on a mammogram picture can be difficult to localise on the breast itself and special techniques have to be used whereby a needle with a curved tip is inserted

16

by a radiologist so that a surgeon is directed accurately to the right area.

It is a disappointment that in women under 35 years changes due to a cancer are difficult to interpret on a mammogram, and so it is not a satisfactory screening test for women in this age range. Even for women between 35 and 50 there is no evidence yet that regular mammogram screening offers any benefit, although mammograms can be useful in individual cases.

Another problem is that not all women who are sent an invitation to attend for a mammogram will do so. In Sweden around 90 per cent of women accept such invitations to screening, but in the UK only around 70 per cent have accepted in previous studies and that is the proportion that is expected to attend the new screening sessions. Reaching the other 30 per cent is going to be difficult.

Occasionally a cancer will fail to show up on a mammogram. Almost as worrying is the fact that sometimes there will be a 'false positive', i.e. a suspicious area shows up on the mammogram but after it has been removed by a minor operation it turns out to be nothing to worry about. However the number of such problems arising is small compared with the benefits of finding early cancers.

The radiation risk of mammograms has worried people. Doesn't exposure to X-rays increase the chances of cancer? Well, the amount of radiation given has been reduced about 15-fold since mammograms were first introduced, and it is now estimated that the risk of any adverse effect on the breast from a mammogram is of the order of one chance in two million.

SHOULD I HAVE A MAMMOGRAM?

The indications for having a mammogram can be summarised as follows.

Aged 50–64
If you are in the age group 50–64 years you should take advantage of the DHSS screening clinics and have a mammogram every three years. Regular mammograms are of proven benefit to you, and it might be better to have more frequent mammograms, perhaps two-yearly, especially if you have lumpy breasts making examination difficult.

If you think you have a lump you need a physical examination as well, so a mammogram is no substitute.

Aged 35–50

If you are in the age group 35–50 years you will not be invited to these new screening sessions and there is no clear evidence that regular screening mammograms are needed. However mammograms should be carried out if a doctor cannot be sure if you have a discrete lump or not, if you have symptoms such as a nipple discharge, or if you are in a high-risk group because of your family history (see Chapter 7) or because you have had a previous breast cancer.

Under 35

If you are under 35 years mammograms are usually no help. Self-examination can be supplemented with ultrasound examination of any doubtful lumpy areas.

Over 64

If you are over 64 years any cancer that forms will tend to be slow-growing and the change in breast tissue that occurs with age will make it easier to feel any lumps. Self-examination and getting problems checked by your doctor will mean that mammograms are only needed if there is a lumpy area that is difficult to be sure about.

Family history is not a risk factor for this age group, but a previous cancer is and means that regular checks are needed, possibly including mammograms.

3

BENIGN PROBLEMS IN THE BREAST

Most breast problems, whether they are lumps or pain, are simple and benign (mild, as opposed to malignant or dangerous). Most are caused by minor alterations in the normal processes that take place in the breast as a result of changes in the circulating hormones. They are not really diseases, just disorders, with hardly any dividing line between normal and abnormal, and they are not serious. They are worrying, however; even if you know they are benign, there is a natural concern that you may be 'prone' to breast problems and that the next problem might be cancer. As we shall see these benign problems usually have no such tendency.

BENIGN MAMMARY DYSPLASIA (BMD)

There are various other names for benign mammary dysplasia – fibroadenosis, chronic mastitis, or fibrocystic disease. It is commonest in women in their 20s and 30s, and many women develop this condition. The main features are lumpiness and breast tenderness. As the pain usually varies with the menstrual cycle, it is often called cyclical mastalgia.

The lumps that occur are difficult to measure because they have ill-defined margins. Both breasts are likely to be affected, especially the upper outer parts. The lumpiness and tenderness vary at different times of the menstrual cycle, and the increasing fluid retention produces an exaggeration of the usual premenstrual tenderness. It may be associated with multiple small cysts in the breasts or with one or more large cysts, up to several centimetres across. Sometimes the lumpiness and tenderness occur separately.

The pain may be just a vague discomfort or it may be severe; it may even produce such tenderness that cuddling children is avoided. It gets worse in the second half of the menstrual cycle and usually goes away completely when the period is over, although sometimes it stays throughout the cycle, getting even worse before the period. In about half the women it is only one breast that is affected. There is a strong association with the other symptoms of premenstrual tension, including headache, irritability and general fluid retention in the body.

The causes seem likely to be hormonal. While it is true that it is not possible to measure any hormonal upset in the blood, the problem does vary with the menstrual cycle, and it disappears after the menopause. It is commoner in women who have had no children, and the more children a woman has had the less likely she is to be troubled by benign mammary dysplasia. It is also less likely to occur in women who are overweight. It is commoner in women who have irregular periods, and is usually reduced by taking the contraceptive pill. Progestogen in the pill is the protective agent, and the longer the pill is taken the greater the protective effect. The hormones prolactin and oestrogen stimulate breast tissue and so are the most likely cause.

There is no clear evidence that women who have benign mammary dysplasia are more likely to get breast cancer, although this was suggested by some earlier studies. However, before any such study can conclude that BMD turns into cancer, it has to be very careful to ensure that all the patients being investigated with benign mammary dysplasia really have this condition, and not the symptoms of early cancers. So, however troublesome pain and lumpiness may be in this condition, as long as you have had a thorough examination to make sure there is no cancer present, you can rest assured that you are not at any increased risk of getting cancer in the future.

Usually the condition just settles of its own accord, although it is always difficult to know whether this is going to take months or years. Often if a woman knows for sure that BMD is the cause of her symptoms it removes her anxiety about cancer and she then notices the symptoms much less.

Treatment for BMD

If the symptoms are severe enough to need treatment, it is

sometimes best to start with dietary changes. Cutting out caffeine from the diet has been claimed to help, but the effect is small and there is some doubt if it even works at all.

Supplementing the essential fatty acids that are an everyday part of the diet is of proven benefit, however, and has very few side effects. This can be done by taking the natural preparation of evening primrose oil in a dose of six 500 mg capsules daily for three months. Evening primrose contains high concentrations of three fatty acids that are a normal part of the diet but play an important role in the functioning of hormones, some of which affect the breast. Evening primrose oil capsules have to be bought in chemists or health-food shops as they are not yet available on prescription.

It probably also helps to cut the intake of saturated fats at the same time (butter, cream, cheese and all other animal fats), because these can interfere with the body's attempts to use these essential fatty acids to manufacture hormones. Vitamin B_6 has often been taken, but on its own it has little effect; it also seems to work by helping the body use the essential fatty acids.

Only a very few women have symptoms so severe that they interfere with work, leisure and family life and need specific medical treatment. Although there are effective treatments available, the reluctance to prescribe them is because they all tend to have some side effects. In the past diuretics (drugs that promote fluid loss from the body) were widely used, but they are not effective and have many undesirable effects on the rest of the body. An effective treatment is the drug danazol which works by suppressing the hormone gonadotrophin. It is given in a dose of 100 mg twice a day and this takes away the pain almost completely in 70 per cent of women. However it does have some troublesome side effects, including headache, weight gain, muscle cramps, irregular periods and an oily skin. Unfortunately when it is stopped there is a tendency for the pain to recur but if it does and there was a good response at first, then continuing danazol in a low dose of 100 mg on alternate days just in the last half of the menstrual cycle is usually effective prevention.

Tamoxifen in a dose of 10 or 20 mg daily takes away the pain in about 80 per cent of women with severe breast pain. It works by blocking the hormone oestrogen. Unfortunately it also has a few side effects, including hot flushes, menstrual irregularity and nausea, although if the dose is kept down to 10 mg daily then only 20 per cent of women get these side effects. The treatment is usually continued for three months. Even more effective is to give bromocriptine in a dose of 2.5 mg twice a day. It takes away the symptoms in up to 90 per cent of women. However it produces even more side effects – nausea, dizziness and headache – although these are minimised by starting the treatment with a low dose and gradually increasing it, most patients not needing more than 5 mg daily. Bromocriptine works by reducing the secretion of the hormone prolactin, and again is usually taken for three months.

Norethisterone, a progestogen taken in a fairly large dose of 5 mg three times a day in the second half of the menstrual cycle, seems to be another effective method of controlling these pains.

So you will see from the above that there are effective treatments available for benign mammary dysplasia, although the drugs used are powerful and need to be carefully supervised. However, none of the drugs has any harmful effects on the breast as far as is known.

CYSTS

A breast cyst is a collection of fluid in the breast. In some cysts the fluid is lymph, in others it is normal secretion from the breast ducts. Usually it is yellow, but sometimes it is brown or green if there has been a little bleeding into the cyst. A cyst may occur in any part of the breast and be any size, from smaller than a pea to greater than 5 cm (2 inches) across. A cyst produces a dome-shaped swelling, usually fairly deep in the breast, that is often tender when it is enlarging. If there are several cysts close together the swelling will be irregular in shape.

Often cysts are a part of benign mammary dysplasia and so tend to occur in the same age range of the 20s and 30s, but they can occur at any age up to the menopause, being rare after that time. What causes them is not clear, but they are not associated in any way with breast cancer or even with a tendency to breast cancer. Sometimes they are clearly due to secretion within a duct; an extreme example of this is a cyst called a galactocele. This contains milk, and occurs in women who have been breastfeeding a few months before. A duct has shrunk down leaving tubules still producing a little milk which blows the duct up into a cyst.

Treatment
If a cyst is found, the first thing to do is to aspirate it. This is done with a syringe and needle and with no anaesthetic, just like taking a blood sample. It is an unpleasant thought having a needle put into the breast, but you feel only a little needle prick. The procedure is quite harmless and is so worthwhile when you see your breast lump being drawn up into the syringe. If there is no remaining lump at all, then you can be certain that it was a benign cyst and tests are not even needed on the fluid to prove this.

If you have had one cyst you are slightly more likely to get another. This can also be aspirated in the same way, and only if they keep recurring persistently would treatment with a drug such as danazol be considered.

DUCT ECTASIA

This is second only to benign mammary dysplasia as a cause of breast pain, and is usually found in women of around 40. It produces breast pain, a lump, nipple discharge and, later on, usually around the 50s, nipple retraction. The nipple discharge is usually milky or watery and may contain recognisable blood or old blood that has turned brown or green.

Within the breast tissue the major ducts dilate and fill with thick milky secretions. These can often be felt as soft irregular-shaped lumps under the edge of the areola. The duct wall then gets inflamed, partly from irritation due to these secretions and also because of infection which gets into the ducts. Occasionally one of the ducts bursts and the body then makes an intense inflammatory reaction to the contents which leak out into the breast, producing a hot, red, painful, swollen and very tender section of the breast. Finally inflammation around the ducts may produce scarring and as the scar tissue contracts it may pull back on the nipple. Despite the pain and discomfort, the condition is quite benign and has no tendency to turn malignant.

23

What causes duct ectasia is not known. It does not seem to be related to previous breastfeeding, as was once suggested. Bacteria are always present in the ducts and they are certainly to blame for most of the complications that occur, but we are not sure whether they start the whole thing off or not. They are usually a particular group of bacteria called anaerobes, meaning they can only flourish in the absence of oxygen, and they respond only to certain antibiotics.

Treatment

Most women with duct ectasia do not need any treatment. As long as your doctor is certain that it is not cancer, it is best to wait and let it settle of its own accord. So far there is little experience of treating the problem with antibiotics; it seems likely that antibiotics that deal with anaerobes might help, although often the problem has progressed to such a stage that they cannot make much difference, and they would probably have to be continued for many months. Metronidazole together with flucloxacillin are the antibiotics usually used together for this condition.

For a very small number of women with troublesome pain, discharge and infection, the condition can be effectively treated by removing the major ducts surgically. Under general anaesthetic a small incision is made around the edge of the areola and a cone of tissue is removed containing all the major ducts as they come up to the nipple.

FIBROADENOMA

A fibroadenoma is a benign breast tumour that has no tendency to turn malignant. It most often occurs in women in their 20s and is discovered as a painless lump. It is usually round and smooth and can be pushed around so easily under the skin that it is known as a 'breast mouse'. It may be the size of a pea when it is first felt and it usually stops growing when it gets to 2 or 3 cm (about an inch) across. It can be in any part of the breast and it is made up of firm white solid tissue.

Treatment

Medicines make no difference to fibroadenomas. It is usually best to remove them, especially as this confirms the diagnosis for certain. It is worrying to go round with a lump in your breast with the constant nagging background thought that something is wrong there. And if a fibroadenoma continues to grow and reaches 3 cm across it produces quite a prominent lump.

The operation itself is very simple, and can usually be done under a local anaesthetic as a day patient (no overnight stay in hospital). Removing a fibroadenoma causes no harm to the breast, will not interfere with subsequent breastfeeding and will not encourage other fibroadenomas to grow. However sometimes in a woman under the age of 25 years, if the diagnosis can be confirmed by a needle biopsy (see page 88) and ultrasound, it is reasonable to wait and watch it and perhaps avoid an operation.

ABSCESS

If an infection gets into the breast tissue it produces inflammation, with redness, pain and swelling. If it progresses for a few days pus may be produced and it then becomes an abscess. When this occurs the painful area throbs and there is often a fever (raised temperature).

The bacteria which most often cause such infections are staphylococci – organisms normally found on the skin surface, where they are harmless. They usually get into the breast tissue through a crack on the edge of the nipple during breastfeeding. If the infection is not related to breastfeeding then it is probably caused by duct ectasia or possibly a cyst that gets infected. It is very rare for it to happen after the menopause.

Treatment

There are several measures that can be taken to prevent cracked nipples in the first place (see Chapter 10). However if you do see signs of infection developing in your breast, with redness and hotness of the skin, you should go to your doctor urgently because if antibiotics active against staphylococci (such as flucloxacillin) are started quickly it may stop an abscess forming.

If the area has been painful for a few days, and particularly if it is throbbing, then it is likely that pus has already formed within it, in which case antibiotics will be no use. Indeed, antibiotics given at this stage can even cause further problems, trapping pus in the abscess so that it appears to settle down but just flares up again later. Instead, an operation to release the pus is needed, under a general anaesthetic – the sooner this is done the quicker it will clear up. You will probably be in hospital for at least one night. After the abscess is opened it will not be stitched up again but left open so that any more pus that forms can be easily removed. Daily dressings will be needed, done either by a district nurse, a nurse at your local surgery or hospital, or by yourself. It is worrying to see an open wound in your breast, and you may wonder if it will ever close and what sort of a giant scar it will leave. However it will close satisfactorily; in fact the problem is to stop it closing too soon, hence the need usually for careful dressings tucked into the wound to keep the edges apart. The subsequent scar will not be a wide round area but a line, albeit sometimes a wide line. There is always a lot of thickening produced in the surrounding breast tissue by an abscess, and this will take months to settle.

Occasionally it is possible to suck out the pus with a wide needle and use antibiotics to destroy the infection, thus avoiding the need for an operation.

DUCT PAPILLOMAS

Like fibroadenomas, duct papillomas are also benign breast tumours, occurring inside the major ducts as little warty projections. Unlike fibroadenomas, however, they have a tendency to turn malignant if left untreated. As they are in the major ducts they will be found close to the nipple and they usually show up first as a bleed from the nipple. The characteristic is that the drop of usually fairly red blood comes each time from the same individual duct on the surface of the nipple. Sometimes it is found that pressure on a certain area at the edge of the areola (over the papilloma) produces this bleeding from the nipple. Duct papillomas only occur in women before the menopause.

Treatment
The treatment is to excise the papilloma – a minor operation performed under a general anaesthetic. An incision is made

26

down the side of the nipple and the individual duct causing the problem is isolated, hopefully with a bulge along it showing where the papilloma is. The duct is then cut out. If there is any doubt about exactly which duct is involved, then all the major ducts are excised, as for duct ectasia, with an incision around the lower edge of the areola.

FAT NECROSIS

This is not a serious condition in any way, although the trauma that produces it usually is. It is important, however, because although it is very rare it produces a lump in the breast that feels exactly like a cancer.

Some minor trauma to the breast – a knock or bump, for example – is an inevitable and everyday occurrence. It does not damage the breast and certainly does not start cancers growing. Fat necrosis, however, is produced by a bang on the breast that is severe enough to cause considerable bruising and to burst open a lot of fat cells. The body does not recognise the released fat as 'self', and reacts violently to it as though it is foreign material. Intense scarring is then produced, making a very firm irregular lump. When all this scar tissue starts to contract, as scar tissue tends to, it pulls on the suspensory ligaments, just as cancer does, producing skin dimpling and a distorted contour of the breast.

If such a lump is found the original trauma will not have been forgotten and so the diagnosis can usually be fairly confident. However if there is the slightest doubt, the lump, like most other breast lumps, should be removed.

4

PROBLEMS YOU MAY DISCOVER IN YOUR BREASTS

'I'VE FOUND A LUMP'

It is easy to get an initial feeling of panic when you find a lump in your breast, and to imagine the worst. You can't believe it could really happen to you. This is often followed by a feeling of regret at not having done a self-examination regularly; now you don't know how long the lump has been there.

The first thing to remember is that the great majority of lumps – around 90 per cent of them – are entirely simple and benign. Check again to see if it is really possible to feel it with the flats of the fingers and not just with the fingertips. If what you are feeling is more the size of a grain of rice than a pea, it is probably of no significance. Also make quite sure it is not a rib by attempting to move it up and down on the chest wall.

Next check to see if it is discrete; that is to say, can you feel where it starts and stops? If you cannot, then check whether it differs from other parts of the breast. Is it different from the same area on the other breast? If it is not different it is probably not a true lump. Often the lower fold of the breast appears to have a ridge along it if the breasts are large and heavy, and this can be mistaken for a lump.

If it is a discrete lump, then it may be one of a number of things, none of them cancer – a fibroadenoma, a cyst, the most prominent part of benign mammary dysplasia, a sebaceous cyst at the edge of the areola, a duct ectasia, or, rarely, a fat necrosis (see Chapter 3 for a description of all these conditions). Or it could be a cancer. If it completely disappears in a few days it must have been fluid and therefore completely safe, benign and needing no treatment.

Whatever it might be, within a week or so of finding a lump you should visit a doctor, preferably your general practitioner. Even if you think it may have gone it is still wise to have it checked.

'I'VE GOT A PAIN IN MY BREAST'

A pain always suggests that some harm is occurring at the site of the pain, and one naturally thinks that something that is painful must be more serious than something that is not painful. However, in general, painful breast lumps are more likely to be benign, while cancer in the breast very rarely causes any pain.

The medical term for breast pain is mastalgia. The pain may be due to benign mammary dysplasia (see pages 19–22) which produces general tenderness that gets worse before periods and then eases when the period starts. This is often called cyclical mastalgia, and may or may not be associated with ill-defined lumpy areas. Although it usually affects both breasts, it may be on one side only, often mainly the upper outer part of the breast. The pain may be caused by many small cysts or by a single larger one. Sometimes there is a locally tender area in the breast, sometimes the pain shoots along the arms as well, and sometimes the pain does not vary with the periods.

Pain may also be caused by duct ectasia (see pages 23–4), especially if a duct bursts inside the breast, producing a very tender and often inflamed area. An abscess also produces pain and a very tender area of the breast that soon leads to redness of the overlying skin. After a while the pain may change to a throbbing.

Occasionally pain that appears to come from the breast in fact comes from somewhere else, such as the ribs, the heart (angina), the lungs, the spine, the muscles of the chest wall or the oesophagus (gullet). Sometimes the pain of shingles is felt in the breast, and only later is it diagnosed when the typical rash appears. Shingles is caused by the chickenpox virus getting into sensory nerves and affecting the area of skin served by the nerves; sometimes in adults it gets into the nerves that run round the chest wall and produces a band of pain, followed days later by a crop of painful blisters.

Breast tenderness is also an early sign of pregnancy; this

29

starts like premenstrual tenderness but increases and persists and leads on to the nipples becoming sensitive.

If you have a pain in the breast you should first check to see if the breast is tender and, second, check to see if there is a lump that you can feel with the flats of the fingers.

- If there is a lump then it should be treated as any other lump – you should contact your doctor.
- Even if there is no lump you should let your general practitioner know about any pain in the breast that persists.

'I'VE GOT A NIPPLE DISCHARGE'

The vast majority of instances of breast discharge are due to simple benign causes.

Such discharge will usually have been first noticed on the clothes – on the inside of your bra, for example. Sometimes it will have been produced by squeezing the nipples, perhaps because they felt tense. You should remember, though, that there is never any need to check for nipple discharge by squeezing your nipples; if the discharge does not come out by itself, it is of no significance.

Discharge may be due to:

- **Duct ectasia** – see pages 23–4. This is the commonest cause. Secretions build up in the ducts, causing irritation. The secretion itself is usually white, creamy or more rarely greenish, but if it produces irritation the duct may weep a watery or even blood-stained fluid.
- **Duct papilloma** – see pages 26–7. Thus is a small wart-like lesion in one of the major ducts that often shows itself by bleeding. The blood always comes from the same duct opening, particularly if pressure is applied over the surface of the papilloma.
- **Hormonal.** This will be particularly likely if levels of the hormone prolactin are high, especially after childbirth. The discharge will be milky and will come from many ducts and usually both nipples. This cause can be confirmed by a blood test (which measures the prolactin level in the blood).
- **Drugs.** Very rarely a discharge can be caused by certain drugs such as those to lower blood pressure, and antidepressant drugs.
- **Cancer.** Probably less than 4 per cent of women with a

30

nipple discharge have cancer, i.e. it is a very rare sign of cancer.

If the discharge is white, creamy or green, and whether it is thin or thick, it is almost certainly due to duct ectasia. If the discharge is blood-stained, or clear and watery, it may also be due to duct ectasia, but can be caused by cancer.

More important than what the discharge looks like is whether it comes from any little ducts on the surface of the nipple or whether it comes from only one. If it is blood-stained and comes from one duct only, especially when one part of the breast near the areola is squeezed, then it is probably due to a benign warty growth in the major ducts, called a duct papilloma.

If you find a nipple discharge on your clothes, always report it to your doctor. What will then be of most concern to your doctor is whether there is a lump under the nipple to feel or to see on a mammogram.

'THERE IS A DIFFERENCE IN BREAST SHAPE OR SKIN DIMPLING'

Often there are differences between the two breasts that have always been present, but it is a recent change that is important. Only if you carry out a regular self-examination will you be able to know what has always been present and what is new.

If there is a recent change in shape, or if skin dimpling occurs, this can be a sign of cancer. This is because a cancer, even when very small, can pull on the suspensory ligaments in the breast and so pull on the skin a long way from where the cancer is situated. It can also pull in on the nipple, even making a previously everted nipple become inverted.

However this sort of change can also be caused by trauma. If a group of fat cells are burst by a hard bang on the breast, a condition called fat necrosis occurs which also produces a hard and irregular lump, very like a cancer. This then pulls on the same suspensory ligaments. However such fat necrosis would always be produced by trauma – a blow or a knock – that you would remember and the bang would certainly have produced a bruise at the time. Old scars from operations can also produce alterations in breast shape or skin dimpling, as

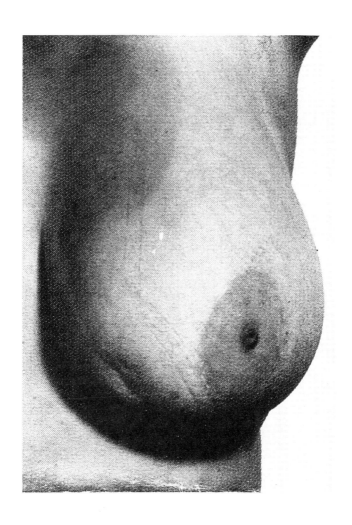

Dimpling of the breast tissue.

can duct ectasia if infection gets into the major ducts and the resulting infection leads to scarring.

'MY BREASTS ARE DIFFERENT SIZES'

Minor differences in size between your breasts are very common – in fact it is almost inevitable that there will be a slight difference.

Occasionally these differences are quite noticeable and may cause embarrassment. Usually this occurs simply because one breast has developed more than the other, but very rarely it can be due to disease within one breast – either an abscess, a cyst, a big benign tumour, or a cancer.

Check first for any lumps or tenderness, particularly if the change seems to be fairly recent. Even if there is no lump, if you are worried about an obvious difference in size of the two breasts you should discuss it with your general practitioner. He will exclude any localised disease and he may refer you to a plastic surgeon with whom you can discuss the possibility of surgical correction of breast sizes (see Chapter 11). If it is the size of both breasts that concerns you, your doctor will also be able to advise if something needs to be done.

'I'VE GOT SORE NIPPLES'

An increasingly common cause of sore nipples is 'jogger's nipple', which occurs as a result of friction between the nipples and clothing when running. The nipples sometimes get so sore that they bleed. Men get this problem as well as women. The treatment is a firmer bra (women) or applying sticky tape over the nipples (both sexes).

Duct ectasia can also cause sore nipples, and when it does it is often associated with nipple discharge.

If the skin of the nipples is red as well as being sore it may be due to eczema, in which case there will usually be similar changes in the skin elsewhere on the body; if not, then it might be the very rare condition of Paget's disease of the nipple, which is caused by an underlying cancer.

Unless the soreness is obviously due to jogging or just part of a generalised eczema, you should consult your doctor.

'THERE ARE CHANGES IN THE SKIN OF THE BREAST'

If there is redness just where the lower part of the breast presses on the chest wall it is probably intertrigo. This skin problem occurs where a fold of skin becomes sweaty and moist; this encourages infection, with ordinary skin-surface bacteria and fungi starting to grow. The skin then gets red and sore because of the infection, the moistness and the rubbing. It commonly occurs underneath the breasts, especially if they are heavy, but can also occur in other places of the body where similar skin folds occur, such as the lower abdomen, umbilicus and groin. The treatment is to stop the two folds of skin rubbing by wearing a firmer bra, and to keep the skin clean and dry by regular daily washing with a skin antiseptic such as Hibiscrub.

Bruises will obviously discolour the skin, but the knock that produced them will usually have been noticed and the colour is usually easily recognised.

Shingles is a viral infection of nerve roots that produces pain at the skin surface and a typical crop of red spots with little scabs in a band round the chest.

Rarely skin changes are from a more serious cause. *Peau d'orange* (French for skin of an orange) is a puffiness of the skin that makes it look like orange peel, and can be caused by infections or by a cancer. Sometimes the skin gets thickened and reddened by a tumour underneath, but in this case there will certainly be a lump that can be felt.

5

WHAT HAPPENS WHEN YOU GET BREAST PROBLEMS INVESTIGATED

Visits to a doctor or a clinic for advice and help on breast problems are particularly worrying if you do not know what is going to happen when you get there or what tests are going to be done or even whether treatment is likely to be started there and then.

VISITS TO YOUR GENERAL PRACTITIONER

If you have any recent change in your breasts, or indeed any breast problem that you want advice on, you should always visit your general practitioner first. He or she will take a history of the problem, ask other questions to help make a diagnosis, and carry out an examination of your breasts by the technique described in Chapter 2. You may find it is a little embarrassing at first, having your breasts inspected and examined, particularly if your doctor is a man. If this bothers you, you can ask for arrangements to be made for an examination by a female doctor.

During the examination the doctor will look for any discrete lump or any other problem that needs further investigation. If the problem is pain it may be found that the cause has nothing to do with the breasts – the problem could lie in the ribs or lungs, for example. If this is the case, it may be possible to give simple treatment there and then.

Depending on what is found, you may be:

- Reassured that no further investigations are needed. This is often because what you felt was not a discrete lump after all, perhaps because you were feeling with the fingertips instead of the flats of the fingers. Often if the problem was breast pain or tenderness, skin changes or even nipple discharge, it is possible that a straightforward examination by your general practitioner can exclude any serious problem.
- Asked to come back again at an interval of some weeks, for review. Often this is because you are being examined in the days just before your period and your general practitioner will want to examine you again at a different time in your menstrual cycle, to see if the lump goes then, in which case the lump will just have been fluid.
- Asked to attend an X-ray clinic for mammograms. Being sent for a mammogram plays no part in deciding how to manage a discrete lump; that will always need a biopsy (see page 38). But you may be sent for a mammogram if there is difficulty in deciding whether or not there is a discrete lump present in a lumpy breast. And if you are in an age group in which it would be good for you to go for a routine screening, you may well be sent for one anyway.
- Referred to a hospital specialist. If you have a lump or any problem that needs further investigations you will be referred to a hospital consultant. However, just because you are given such a referral does not necessarily mean that something is wrong and you have a breast 'disease'. A general practitioner deals with the whole spectrum of problems, from infancy to old age, from haemorrhoids to heart attacks, and cannot be an expert in everything. So it may well be that you are just being referred for a further opinion, and this may well show that there is no problem and that nothing further needs to be done.

VISITS TO A HOSPITAL SPECIALIST

In some countries it is the gynaecologist who deals with breast problems, but in the UK this work is performed by consultant general surgeons. However, you must not think that because they are surgeons they can only deal with breast problems by the use of surgery. Nor is it the case that, because they see patients with other problems, they do not have specialist experience of dealing with breast problems. You will be seen by someone who regularly deals with breast problems and who will be familiar with the latest treatments.

Before going to a hospital specialist you will have to have a referral letter from your general practitioner; it will either be given to you to take with you or it will be sent direct to the specialist. You can ask to go to a particular specialist if you wish, but your GP is best placed from previous experience to know which of the specialists at your local hospital will be best able to help you.

The aim is that you will get an appointment within a week or two, see the consultant personally rather than one of the other members of the team, and that all staff you come in contact with should be well aware of the anxiety that breast problems cause. Unfortunately no system is perfect, so you might have to wait longer for an appointment, and you might not get to see the consultant personally. It is to be hoped, though, that the staff you do see will be sympathetic to your anxieties. When you do get to the clinic the waiting time should be kept to a minimum, but it may be wise to take a paper or a book.

Many women worry that they may be 'wasting the specialist's time' by going along with a lump that they are not sure is real, or that has recently disappeared or with symptoms that are only mild. You should never think that. You can be sure that the specialist will be as delighted as you if your breast problem turns out to be something that is not serious and can be rapidly resolved.

The specialist will want you to repeat again the details of what you have noticed and when it first started, and will also want to ask a variety of questions about your breasts and other aspects of your health, past and present. There will then be an examination of your breasts and probably other areas such as your neck, abdomen, heart and lungs.

Tests

Some tests may be done there and then in the clinic. If your problem is a breast lump and the examination suggests that it is a cyst, it will be aspirated (drawn up into a syringe, see page 23) and that will be the end of it.

37

If the lump is not a cyst but is solid, then, after an explanation is given of what needs to be done, a needle biopsy may be taken in the clinic. This is usually done with a thin blood-taking needle and a syringe, and it feels much the same as having a blood sample taken from your arm. The needle is inserted into the lump in your breast, a little fluid containing a few cells is sucked out of the lump, the needle is removed and the fluid and cells are squirted onto a microscope slide. The cells from the lump will subsequently be examined microscopically to determine its precise nature.

Occasionally a wider needle is used to get a core of tissue, and for this a local anaesthetic will be given; however it still only takes about three minutes and is done in the outpatient clinic. Both techniques can lead to a little bruising in the breast but this is of no significance and will clear (although it will be tender for a few days) and the procedure itself is quite safe. Sometimes it is decided to go straight to an excision biopsy (a minor operation to remove the lump), without a needle biopsy.

Blood tests may be taken in the clinic. If you have already had mammograms carried out the specialist can look at them in the clinic. If not you may have to have these done in the X-ray department, either that day or a few days later.

What the consultant will tell you
Even on your first visit it may be possible for the specialist to give you a fairly full account of what is the cause of your symptoms and what the treatment will be, although this may not be possible if you are having further tests done. It usually takes a few days to get the results of a needle biopsy, so in that case you will be given a further appointment to discuss all the results of the tests.

Do ask all the questions you want to – make a list of questions beforehand, to help you remember everything – and in particular ask about anything that has not been made clear to you. Often all sorts of important questions will occur to you after you have left. If you have another appointment you can of course ask them next time; if not, you can get back in touch with the specialist by letter or phone, or alternatively ask your GP. Everything happens rather quickly in a consultation, particularly when such important matters are to be decided. Some women prefer to go in to the consultation with their husband or another relative or with a friend, and certainly you are always welcome to do this. They may be able to remind you of questions you had wanted to ask, and it can also make you feel a lot less defenceless.

What happens next?
So, after the consultation it is to be presumed that you will:
- Have received an assurance that the problem is simple and needs no further treatment or investigation.
- Have received satisfactory treatment there in the clinic.
- Have had further investigations arranged with another appointment.
- Have had arrangements made for admission to hospital for tests or an operation.

If your breast lump was not a cyst and your specialist thought it was benign, he or she may not have done a needle biopsy but just arranged to get you directly into hospital to have it removed. If it is thought that the lump is a fibroadenoma, for instance, it is still likely that it will need to be removed, even if a needle biopsy confirms it is benign. Nearly always if the specialist confirms it is a discrete lump it is going to have to be removed anyway; this involves a small incision, the lump goes, and this minor operation causes no harm to the rest of the breast. It may be done under a general anaesthetic, but sometimes just a local anaesthetic is used, in which case you will be admitted as a day patient with no overnight stay in hospital.

If you are admitted to hospital to have the lump excised, then that is all there is to it. There will always be the opportunity to discuss the need for any other operation later, if for instance subsequent tests did show that the lump was cancer after all.

VISITS TO AN X-RAY DEPARTMENT FOR A MAMMOGRAM

For the new DHSS-arranged screening clinics, women aged 50–64 years will get letters from their GPs inviting them to attend. There will be no examination, so if you happen to have found a lump in your breast or to have some other breast symptom, this screening is no substitute for seeing your general practitioner about it. For these screening mammograms a

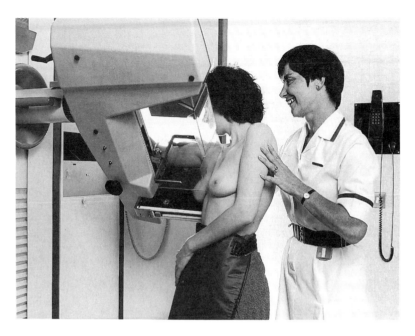
Mammography being performed.

single oblique film will be taken of each breast; on other occasions the standard two films are done on each breast.

For a mammogram you will have to undress to the waist and stand up close to the X-ray machine. The two views are taken first from the side, and then from the top, with the breast pressed down onto a plate; this can be uncomfortable, especially if the breast is small.

The person who takes the X-ray is called a radiographer. While the X-ray is being taken he or she stands behind a screen, and you might be concerned that the radiographer is so well screened from the effects of the X-rays while you get no such protection at all. However, you will probably only have one or two X-rays in a year and thus be exposed to a minimal amount of radiation, whereas a radiographer may do thousands of X-rays during that time and so could potentially be exposed to a large amount of radiation, if it wasn't for the screening.

You will not be given any results there and then because the X-ray films take a while to process and then have to be examined carefully and thoroughly by a consultant radiologist who issues a report a day or so later.

Especially if you have had a single oblique view taken of each breast, do not be alarmed if you are recalled for further films. We know from studies already completed that, after screening with a single oblique film, approximately 10 women in every 100 will need to be recalled. These 10 will then have further films taken, on this occasion the standard top and side views. After that seven of the 10 will be found to have no abnormality, while the other three out of the 100 will be advised to see a hospital specialist, who will probably recommend a biopsy.

6

THE BREASTS DURING PREGNANCY AND BREASTFEEDING

PREGNANCY

Early in pregnancy the breasts prepare themselves for the task of feeding the baby after delivery. Indeed the changes occur so early that tenderness is one of the first signs of pregnancy, noticeable from about the fifth week. Luckily this discomfort does not usually last more than a few weeks. At around the sixth week the little sebaceous glands (Montgomery's tubercles) in the areola become prominent; they produce a lubricant which helps to keep the nipple supple.

By the eighth week the areola begins to darken, and continues to do so throughout the pregnancy. This effect is less noticeable in fairskinned women. Some of the pigmentation fades after delivery, but the areola will always remain darker than it was before the pregnancy.

By 16 weeks a clear liquid called colostrum may be secreted. This is important during early breastfeeding, and will be mentioned in more detail later (see page 46). Little crusts may form as it dries; these can be gently washed off using warm water – soap may be an irritant and is best avoided.

The breasts increase in size throughout pregnancy, and will generally each weigh about 1½ pounds (0·7 kg) more than before. This is due to the increase in glandular tissue and in the number of milk ducts, in preparation for breastfeeding. A larger and more supportive bra will not only be more comfortable, but will also help to prevent unnecessary stretching and then sagging of the breasts later. There is only a certain amount of elasticity in the skin and underlying tissues, so stretch marks are more likely to occur if weight is put on rapidly early in pregnancy. This is one reason for not over-eating in pregnancy. These stretch marks will fade, but are unlikely to disappear completely.

The veins under the skin become more prominent, as there is an increased blood supply to the tissues. The nipples also undergo a number of changes. They become softer and more prominent, so that the baby can grip more easily during feeding. Even flat or slightly inverted nipples are usually prominent by the end of the pregnancy. Sometimes however this fails to occur, and may be a problem when trying to breastfeed. Nipple shields can help to overcome this. They are made of rubber, plastic or glass, are dome-shaped, and have a hole in the middle through which the nipple is pressed. They are used after delivery by women whose nipples still remain inverted and are worn for a short time before feeding, to encourage the nipples to protrude.

BREASTFEEDING

Breastfeeding has so many advantages that it is difficult to believe that bottle-feeding was once so strongly advocated and fashionable. Each species of mammal has its own special type of milk, which differs from all the others and is uniquely suited to its own kind; formula milk can never be as advantageous to babies as breastmilk (and cow's milk should not be used for babies under six months).

So what are the advantages of breastfeeding?

Advantages for the mother

Breastfeeding makes bonding (the development of a close relationship between mother and baby) easier. The physical contact between them is closer during breastfeeding than bottle-feeding, and it also tends to take longer than bottle-feeding. And the breastfeeding mother is likely to spend more time with her baby generally, simply because she cannot easily rely on other people to feed it. If possible, for the greatest success in both breastfeeding and bonding, the baby should be put to the breast within 12 hours of delivery.

Breastfeeding is also the easiest way to lose the weight gained during pregnancy. Although lactating women are advised to eat more (an extra 500 calories is often recom-

43

mended), nevertheless they lose weight. Interestingly, research has shown that the majority of women do not eat as much as advised, and yet neither they nor their babies suffer. The body seems to use food more efficiently during lactation, so less food is needed than originally thought.

Breastmilk does not need preparing or sterilising, and is always 'on tap'. This is particularly useful when travelling, visiting friends, and feeding in the middle of the night. There is less embarrassment about breastfeeding nowadays, but if necessary it is usually possible to find some privacy in which to feed. And remember, it is relatively easy to change from breastfeeding to the bottle, but the reverse is not true, so persevere if you can.

Advantages for the baby
Breastmilk provides a perfectly balanced food, ideally suited to a baby's requirements. Even the best formula milks cannot completely match the composition of breastmilk, which contains not only the correct nutritional requirements but always in the right concentrations. It is quite easy to put in too much powder when making up a bottle, and this can lead to dehydration if the baby is not offered water as well.

Antibodies (part of the body's immune defences) which a woman has made to previous infections pass into her milk, and so she is able to pass on some of this protection to her baby; for example, breastfed babies are less likely to suffer from gastroenteritis (tummy upsets) and coughs and colds. Studies have also shown there are fewer cot deaths in breastfed babies, but we do not know the reasons for this yet. Additionally, breastfed babies are less likely to develop eczema and allergies to cow's milk and eggs than bottle-fed ones, although these problems can still occur even in breastfed babies, particularly if the parents are prone to these conditions. It has been suggested that mothers can make it less likely that they will pass this susceptibility on to the baby by avoiding eggs and cow's milk themselves while lactating.

Babies on breastmilk are less likely to be overweight than those on formula milk. This has advantages in later life, as excessively heavy babies tend to grow into overweight adolescents and adults. Breastfed babies do gain weight very fast, especially in the first few weeks, when the milk supply is more than they really need, but they grow in length as well, and so stay nicely in proportion.

In conclusion, the breast is ideally adapted for all the baby's needs: it is soft and comfortable; it produces a perfectly-balanced, totally-comprehensive feed, at the right temperature. Of course, advantages for the baby are indirectly advantages for the mother, and vice versa. A healthy, happy baby is much easier to look after, and will give more pleasure to both parents, and a happy and relaxed mother will tend to have a more contented baby.

WHAT DOES BREASTFEEDING ACTUALLY INVOLVE?

Unfortunately, the picture is not always so rosy. Breastfeeding can be very traumatic at first, when the mother is getting over the delivery, getting to know the baby and its demands, and often having to run a home as well. Also some babies are not as easy to cope with as others, and some women are actually repelled by the idea of breastfeeding; if this is so, they should not be made to feel guilty or failures.

There is no denying that breastfeeding involves a major commitment on the part of both parents. To be successful, feeding must be more or less on demand, night and day. This means the mother is unlikely to be able to go out to work, and the father may be going to work after a disturbed night. Ideally the whole question should be thought out during the pregnancy, so that by the time the baby arrives on the scene, all advantages and disadvantages have been weighed up and a decision made. Any preparations should have been made beforehand, so that as little as possible needs to be organised at the last minute.

A book of this size, dealing with many other aspects of the breasts, cannot give a full discussion of breastfeeding. However, the points made here should act as a guide, and you will find more detailed information in the books listed under Further Reading.

At the beginning
It is important that the baby is put to the breast as soon as possible after delivery, and certainly within 12 hours. Some babies start to suck right away, but others may be slower; for

example, if pethidine is given to the mother for pain relief during labour the baby will also be affected by it and may be a bit too sleepy at first.

During the first few days, colostrum is produced by the breasts. This looks thinner and less nourishing than 'proper' milk, but in fact it is very important because it contains the antibodies which protect the baby against infection (and which are not present in formula milks). Even if you do not continue to breastfeed, it is worth while perservering for the first few days to give the baby the benefit of this protection.

After a few days, full milk production begins. At each feed, the first milk (called 'fore milk') looks watery, and some mothers worry that it is not strong enough to nourish the baby. Fortunately it is followed by the thicker creamier-looking 'hind milk'.

The 'let-down reflex'

When the baby sucks on the nipple, a reflex release of two hormones occurs, called oxytocin and prolactin. Oxytocin causes muscles to contract, in particular those around the milk ducts, resulting in a good flow of milk. Oxytocin also makes the muscle of the uterus (womb) contract, and is the cause of the so-called 'after pains' which occur particularly during breastfeeding; although painful, they result in the uterus contracting down to its normal size more quickly. The release of oxytocin, which allows milk to flow freely, is called the 'let-down reflex'.

Oxytocin, in its turn, stimulates the production of the second hormone, prolactin, by the pituitary gland at the base of the brain. Prolactin, as its name suggests, is in charge of milk production; the more the nipple is stimulated, the more prolactin is produced, and so more milk is produced. This is why frequent feeding is necessary if breastfeeding is to be successful, and why milk production falls if the baby is given too many supplementary bottle-feeds. It is best to avoid giving extra bottle-feeds if at all possible, as sometimes the breasts stop producing milk altogether.

The let-down reflex may also be inhibited if the mother is anxious or under stress. If this happens only the thin 'fore milk' will appear, and the baby will not be satisfied. It is then easy for a vicious circle to occur, with the mother getting even more anxious as the baby goes on crying. It is therefore important

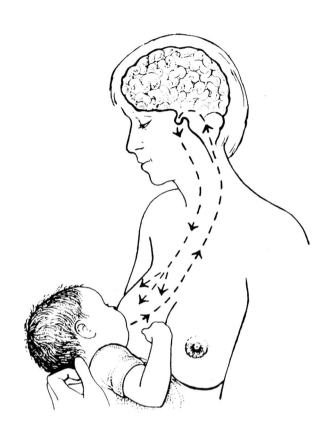

The 'let-down reflex'.

to try and start off in a relaxed frame of mind, in a quiet room, with as much privacy as possible.

Positioning the baby

It is important that both mother and baby are comfortable. The baby must be in a position to hold the nipple correctly, or soreness and cracking may occur. The whole nipple and areola should be inside the baby's mouth. This means that when the baby closes its mouth, its gums press on the milk ducts nearest the surface and this stimulates the flow of milk.

47

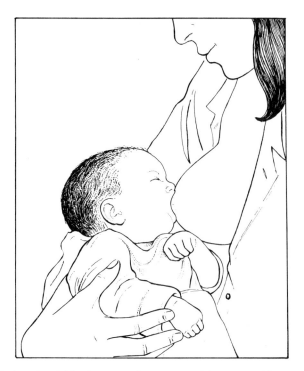

The baby should be in a comfortable position to suckle properly.

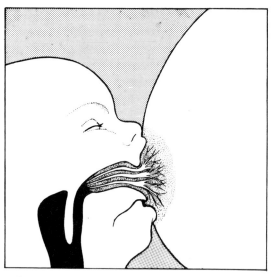

The whole of the nipple and areola should be inside the baby's mouth.

How often should you feed your baby?

The simple answer to this is 'As often as the baby wants to be fed'. As we have seen, the more frequently the nipple is stimulated, the better the milk production. You can even put the baby to the breast when it is not obviously hungry, as suckling gives comfort as well as food. In general, after the first few weeks, the baby wants to be fed less often so the strain of demand feeding decreases naturally.

TAKING MEDICATION WHILE BREASTFEEDING

In general, all forms of medication should be avoided if possible while breastfeeding, since relatively little is known about their effects on the baby. Certain common drugs are secreted into breastmilk, including some sedatives, iodide-containing cough mixtures, and cold remedies containing ephedrine or pseudoephedrine. However there is no need to deny yourself a simple painkiller (preferably paracetamol) when you have a splitting headache. Similarly, if you need antibiotics, you can usually continue breastfeeding, but make sure you check with your doctor. Some medicines, though, can be harmful to the baby if enough passes into the breastmilk and so you should not breastfeed if you need to take them. They include drugs used in thyroid disorders, in the treatment of cancer, and ergotamine, which is used in the treatment of migraine. It is a good rule always to check with your doctor or pharmacist before you take any kind of medication, both during pregnancy and lactation.

The combined oral contraceptive pill is not recommended during breastfeeding because it contains oestrogen which tends to suppress lactation. However, you can take the progestogen-only pill; this contains no oestrogen, is considered safe for the baby, and does not interfere with the milk supply. It contains only a tiny dose of progestogen, of which virtually none enters the milk; it has been calculated that if the baby is breastfed for two years, it will only have taken the equivalent of one tablet during that whole time.

49

THE EFFECTS OF ALCOHOL AND SMOKING

Both alcohol and smoking should be avoided. If you drink, alcohol will be present in your breastmilk in the same concentration as in your blood, so if you are over the limit, your baby may be too. Having said that, the odd drink is harmless, but heavy drinking is known to affect the baby's development. Heavy drinking may also inhibit the let-down reflex.

Smoking, apart from all its other bad effects, reduces milk production, and so should be avoided.

CLOTHES DURING BREASTFEEDING

In general, clothes are likely to become stained when looking after a young baby, whether or not you are breastfeeding. There are a few practicalities worth bearing in mind, however.

For example, dresses which do up at the back will be impractical, since you may need help to undo them before you can breastfeed. And the same applies to bras. Front-fastening maternity bras are available, with flaps which open separately for each cup. In addition, leaking of milk can occur, either between feeds or from the breast that is not being used, so you may need to put what are called 'nursing pads' into each cup.

PROBLEMS WHICH MAY OCCUR DURING BREASTFEEDING

Engorgement

This commonly occurs in the first week. The breasts become swollen, lumpy, tender and hot, due to a build-up of milk in the breasts. This increases the pressure on the milk ducts, causing them to leak tissue fluid, further increasing the pressure. If this process is not halted, breastfeeding will fail.

As with most things, prevention is better than cure. The easiest way to prevent the breasts becoming engorged is to feed the baby frequently. This prevents overfilling.

Once engorgement has occurred, the same applies. Empty the breasts as much and as often as possible. Feed the baby even when it does not appear to be hungry, and try to feed for longer periods.

Sometimes the breasts are so tense and tender that feeding is painful and difficult. If this is the case, try expressing a little milk by hand, or using a breast pump. There is a variety of breast pumps available, either worked by hand or electricity. They are often expensive to buy, but can be rented from the National Childbirth Trust, the La Leche League and other organisations. Alternatively your community midwife or local hospital will usually be able to lend you one, and are always there to help if you have problems.

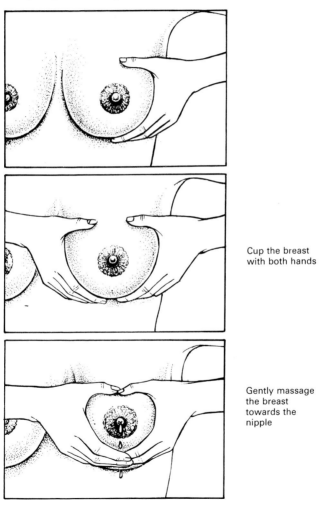

Cup the breast with both hands

Gently massage the breast towards the nipple

Expressing milk by hand.

51

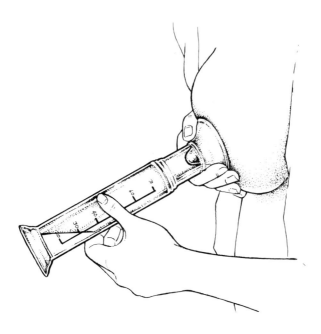

Expressing milk using a breast pump.

A hot bath may encourage leakage of milk, and a simple painkiller may relieve the pain enough to permit feeding. Pain can also be relieved using ice packs or compresses or by splashing the breasts with water.

Sore or cracked nipples

Most mothers who breastfeed will have sore nipples at some time, some worse than others. Although the last thing you will want to do then is feed from the breast, you should continue to do so or your supply will dry up. Once again, prevention is better than cure; there are several factors which predispose to sore nipples, and you should try to avoid these.

Babies who are fed to a schedule are more likely to be very hungry and will therefore suck more strongly, causing soreness. Frequent feeding prevents this. Positioning the baby's mouth is also important. The whole of the areola, not just the nipple, should be in the baby's mouth. If not, then it will chew on the nipple, making it sore. And try to vary the baby's position during feeds so as to spread the load, so that even pressure is applied all round the areola.

Nipples which are continually moist are liable to become sore. Try to leave the breasts exposed to the air as much as possible, as this will help to keep them dry. Cotton bras are better than synthetic ones, as they absorb moisture and allow it to evaporate to a greater extent. Similarly, change bra pads frequently so that they don't get too wet. Some women find it helpful to let a little milk dry on the surface of the nipple after a feed, forming a protective covering. Various barrier creams and sprays are available, and can be soothing, but do not use soap or detergents on the delicate nipple skin. When the skin is already sensitive it is more likely to react to biological washing powders, so these should be avoided as well.

Pain or fear of pain may inhibit the let-down reflex, causing a vicious circle as the baby becomes hungry and sucks more strongly. It will not do any harm to take a simple painkiller before feeding. Also make sure you are warm and comfortable. Usually one breast is less sore, and should be offered first. Hopefully, by the time the sore breast is being used, milk should be flowing freely and less suction will be needed.

If the problem is being caused by poorly protractile nipples, wearing a nipple shield for a short time before feeding may help to make the nipples stand out more. This makes it easier for the baby to suck.

Sometimes a sore nipple actually cracks and may bleed. If this occurs, you may need to stop using that breast for a couple of days, but you should continue to express milk and feed it to the baby with a spoon, providing there is no blood in the milk. Avoid letting the baby get used to a bottle.

Soreness and cracks can also be caused by a yeast infection, known as thrush. The baby can pick it up during birth, as it is very common in the vagina. Thrush in the baby's mouth produces white patches that cannot, unlike curds of milk, be scraped off, and it needs to be treated with antifungal drops, which your doctor can prescribe. The ones most commonly used contain nystatin. You should use an antifungal cream yourself on the breast skin.

Blocked duct and mastitis

A blocked duct is in many ways similar to engorgement, but on a smaller scale. A milk duct becomes blocked, perhaps due to pressure from an ill-fitting bra, and the stagnant milk behind it increases the pressure, causing a lump. Each time you feed, the milk production increases the pressure, making the lump more painful. Despite this, the way to treat the condition is to breastfeed as frequently as possible. If it is allowed to progress, inflammation and then infection will develop. Once it gets to this stage the condition is known as mastitis. However, if you take steps at the first sign of a blocked duct, the problem can be solved quite simply and easily.

The most important thing is to keep emptying the breast as much as and as often as possible. Even when the baby has finished feeding, express milk until the breast is empty. This relieves the pressure. Massage the lump towards the nipple both during and after a feed. Vary the baby's position on the breast at each feed. Bathe the breast with hot water, or use a hot-water bottle. If inflammation is present, you may feel feverish, in which case there is no harm in taking an occasional aspirin, or paracetamol.

If there has been no marked improvement within 24 hours, see your doctor as you will need a course of antibiotics. It is important not to delay treatment, or a generalised breast infection or an abscess may develop.

If you do develop an infection, the breast will become red, hot, swollen and painful, and the skin will look shiny. Usually, despite the antibiotics, you can continue to breastfeed, although if the infection becomes more serious you will be advised not to feed from the infected breast. However you should still continue to express milk from that breast, even though it will not be used. You can feed the baby from the other breast.

Breast abscess

This tends to develop if mastitis is not treated correctly, and is more likely to develop if you stop feeding or expressing milk. Antibiotics will be needed, but in addition surgical drainage of the abscess may be necessary.

Milk retention cyst (galactocele)

A galactocele is a non-tender lump which sometimes occurs following a blocked duct, though this may not be obvious. It is a cyst which becomes filled with milk. Sometimes the cyst can be drained just by massaging the lump towards the nipple. If this does not work, it will need to be removed surgically or infection may develop and cause an abscess.

BABIES WITH SPECIAL DIFFICULTIES

Babies may be affected by pethidine given to the mother for pain relief during labour. They may be more drowsy than is usual, and so will not start to suckle immediately. This is a setback, but can be overcome by persistence. If the baby will not suck, express the milk and give it on a spoon. Avoid using bottles, or the baby will not breastfeed well later. This problem usually does not last more than a couple of days.

Premature babies and very small babies are a special problem. They may not yet have developed a sucking reflex, so they will not feed well at the breast. The more premature the baby, the longer it will take before it can suck. However, these babies are particularly in need of the protection against infection which colostrum and breastmilk provide. You can express milk using a breast pump just as frequently as if you were actually breastfeeding, and the milk can then be fed to the baby by spoon or by a tube. With luck, the baby will be able to breastfeed normally when it is big enough.

Such babies who are bottle-fed at the start sometimes find it much more difficult to change over and feed from the breast. This is because the rubber teat is an easier source of milk than the breast – it requires less work on the part of the baby to obtain the milk. Once it has discovered the rubber teat, it will be less inclined to put in the effort needed at the breast and at having to learn a new technique of sucking. This is why, if breastfeeding is not possible for a while, it is better to feed with a spoon rather than a bottle.

Some babies are either too ill to, or cannot, suck, for example because of infection or a congenital abnormality such as a cleft palate. It is then possible for the mother to express her milk regularly and for it to be fed to the baby by tube. If she cannot produce enough milk in this way herself, some hospitals have a system whereby mothers with extra milk express it and it is then used to augment the supply.

HOW LONG SHOULD YOU GO ON BREASTFEEDING?

The simple answer to this is 'For as long as you like'. There are no hard and fast rules. As mentioned earlier, even if you breastfeed for only the first few days, this will be valuable to your baby because of the anti-infective properties of colostrum.

It is generally agreed that if possible you should try to breastfeed for at least three months, and six months would be even better. This gives the baby the optimum food during the important early months, and helps to protect it from the foreign proteins which can cause allergies.

Although breastfeeding for longer than six months is unusual in this country, that does not mean it is undesirable. If you and your baby are happy to continue, you should do so.

WEANING AND SUPPRESSION OF LACTATION

When you wish to wean the baby, gradually replace breast-feeds with solids, cow's milk (after six months) and fruit juices so that the baby takes less and less milk from the breast. As the stimulus to milk production becomes weaker, the supply will gradually and painlessly diminish. Sometimes the baby finds the breast so soothing that it merely sucks for comfort, especially at bedtime. It is sometimes a difficult habit to break, but it can be done, although it may need a lot of patience.

Suppression of lactation, either after delivery, or if breast-feeding has to stop suddenly, is done simply by inducing a state of engorgement. A tight bra is worn and feeding is stopped. The pressure caused by the milk in the ducts halts the production of more milk, so other measures, such as drugs like bromocriptine, are only rarely necessary.

FINALLY

Most problems with breastfeeding can be overcome, with the correct treatment and a lot of patience. Advice is available from various sources. Midwives and health visitors are specially trained to give advice and support when they do their routine home visits, and GPs and clinic doctors are also there to help. Friends and relations are not always so useful; breastfeeding was not fashionable in our parents' generation, and they may not have the necessary experience.

There are two organisations which actively promote breast-feeding, the National Childbirth Trust and the La Leche

League, both of whom produce a lot of literature, have a network of counsellors and classes, and organise social events. Their addresses are given at the back of the book.

Lactation is the prime function for which the breasts were actually designed. We are the only species in whom the breasts have also taken on a sexual role, and, unfortunately, it is often this aspect which is viewed as the more important. Breastfeeding does not result in ugly breasts if proper care is taken during pregnancy and feeding, and so a mother who breastfeeds need not worry that she will 'lose her figure'. A woman who wants to feed her baby herself should feel confident that it will be a positive experience, both for herself and her baby.

7

EFFECT OF THE PILL AND OTHER HORMONES

CONTRACEPTIVE PILLS

There are two kinds of contraceptive pill.
- One contains two hormones, oestrogen and progestogen, and is called the combined oral contraceptive pill (COC).
- The other contains only progestogen without any oestrogen and is called the progestogen-only pill (POP).

The COC is what most people refer to as 'the pill' and the POP is sometimes referred to as the 'mini-pill'. The term mini-pill is misleading, however, because the POP is not a low-dose version of the COC; it is actually a quite different type of pill, with a different mechanism of action, different side effects and different health risks. It should therefore be assessed on its own, and not in conjunction with the COC.

CHANGES IN THE BREAST CAUSED BY THE COC

Women often experience some breast tenderness and swelling in the first few months after starting the COC. In the vast majority this will disappear within three months. The oestrogen in the COC causes the breast tissue to become more active, just as in early pregnancy; indeed one of the first signs of pregnancy is breast tenderness, often with enlargement.

If the breast tenderness persists after three or four months, a change of brand may help. COCs are described as being oestrogen-dominant or progestogen-dominant, depending on their formulation, and although these are very loose terms, they do reflect their behaviour as regards side effects.

58

COCs which are oestrogen-dominant are more likely to cause persistent breast tenderness or swelling. In such cases, a brand should be chosen which is more progestogen-dominant. Triphasic COCs, in which the dose of hormones varies during the month, seem to give rise to breast tenderness in the last week of the packet. Many women accept this as normal premenstrual tenderness and therefore find it unremarkable, or take vitamins and other preparations to try to control it. However the problem can often be dealt with simply by changing to a monophasic COC, in which the dose of hormones is the same throughout the packet. If you think about it, premenstrual symptoms should not occur on the COC, since ovulation, and hence true periods, are abolished. (The bleeding which occurs in the pill-free week is simply a response to the sudden withdrawal of the hormones.)

Experience has shown that different women will have different reactions to COCs, and it may even take a couple of changes before the best formulation is found for a particular individual.

THE COC AND BENIGN (NON-MALIGNANT) BREAST PROBLEMS

It has been shown that COC users are less likely to suffer from most types of benign breast problems. These include fibroadenomas and cysts, both of which are common in young women. Obviously, such a protective effect is an advantage, since all lumps are worrying and may lead to unnecessary investigations and operations. The protection is thought to be due to the progestogen component of the COC, so if you have a tendency to these problems, you will be best suited to a progestogen-dominant COC, as explained above.

THE COC AND BREAST CANCER

Since the late 1970s there has been an increasing stream of research papers on this subject appearing in the medical press. Unfortunately the lay press chooses to highlight only those studies which have shock value, and usually disregards, or plays down, any studies which are reassuring. It is not surprising, therefore, that many women are confused about the pill and cancer. The truth – or rather what we know of it – is much more complicated.

Before we enter into any discussion about the various studies, one basic fact should be made clear. All the papers to date have concentrated on women who took high-dose COCs. The doses used in the past were two or three times as high as those in the current low-dose combined pills, which have only been in use since about 1981. Effects that occur when women are taking high-dose pills cannot be extrapolated to women taking these low-dose pills.

One of the other major problems which besets all the studies is that the cause, or causes, of breast cancer are still unknown. All we know for certain is that there are a number of associated risk factors, for example late age at first full-term pregnancy, and these risk factors have to be taken into account when assessing the risk due to the COC. The result is that it is not possible to be sure that the women on the COC who show a raised incidence of breast cancer do not also have some other unknown risk factor.

There are thus many problems involved in the construction of research projects, so when you see an article telling you the results of the latest study, whatever it is, you should be aware that the data and results can only be interpreted once you know how the work was actually done. It can be very difficult to interpret such statistics.

This leads us on to the subject of statistics. Another important feature of any research is the number of women in the study. If only a small number are looked at, it is easy for results to be biased. All other things being equal, the larger the number of women in the study, the more reliable it is.

One of the most prominent features of the research in this area is that the studies are forever contradicting one another. One year a paper is published which suggests that there is an increased risk, the next year (or even the same year) another shows there is no increased risk. Heated arguments develop between the experts in the field. Which was the better study? Which one was bigger? Are there any obvious causes of bias? What about the statistics? And so on.

For example, there has been a study which showed that women on the COC presented earlier with their breast cancer and had better survival rates. This may be because they are more likely to be seeing a doctor regularly, and are therefore more likely to have breast examinations, either by the doctor or as a result of being taught self-examination. It has also been suggested that perhaps the hormones in the COC somehow slow down the growth or spread of a tumour.

In contrast, there have been a number of small studies which have shown an increased risk of breast cancer, particularly in young women on the COC. The one which received the most publicity tried to relate the increase in risk to the type of progestogen in the COCs being used (there are several different types in use). This study looked at just over 300 women under the age of 37 who developed breast cancer and who had taken the COC. They found that there was an increased risk of breast cancer if the COC had been taken for more than four years before the age of 25. They also showed that the risk varied with the type of progestogen. This paper was published in 1983, received extensive media coverage, and caused a mass panic among both women taking the COC and the doctors prescribing it. It was subsequently shown, however, that the assessment of progestogens was quite wrong, and that the way in which the research had been carried out made other errors likely. As usual, however, its fall from grace received nothing like the original publicity.

Another small study, which was published in 1986, showed an increased risk if the COC had been taken for more than eight years before the first full-term pregnancy. The correspondence relating to this study was published in a leading medical journal; it ran for six months, becoming increasingly heated, increasingly personal and more and more complicated. The very fact, however, that such a storm arose suggests that it should be viewed with some caution. In the same year, indeed in the same week, a second study of a similar size was published, showing no increase in risk with either time or duration of use. (The above-mentioned caustic correspondence was not actually between the two groups involved in these studies.)

We have given these few illustrations to show just how difficult it is to make any judgment. However, a third paper, also published in 1986 at about the same time, was more reassuring. This study looked at over 4,000 women with breast cancer. In terms of size, this was bigger than all the other studies put together. It was a very careful and well thought-out piece of research, of which few criticisms have been made. It showed no increase in risk with age, type of progestogen, nor with duration of use before the first full-term pregnancy. Indeed, it showed no increase in risk with even 15 years of use of the COC. At the present time, this study is the most convincing. Indeed, Professor Martin Vessey, an epidemiologist, has described it as 'the largest and perhaps the best of the published epidemiological investigations' and has recommended that 'it would seem reasonable for clinical practice to continue to be shaped by the findings in this study unless and until there is equally pressing evidence to the contrary' (*International Planned Parenthood Federation Medical Bulletin*, December 1987). However, we still don't have enough research on long term pill use before a first full-term pregnancy, and the risk of developing breast cancer in later life.

What does all this mean in terms of normal daily life? It means that, on balance, the evidence at present is against an increased risk of breast cancer due to COC use. However, it is advisable to use low-dose pills whenever possible. Further research is needed, particularly to look at women on low-dose formulations and use before a full-term pregnancy. The results will be awaited with great interest.

THE POP AND BREAST PROBLEMS

As mentioned at the beginning of this chapter, the progestogen-only pill (POP) is quite different from the combined pill (COC). It contains no oestrogen at all, and its dose of progestogen is only one-third of that in the COC.

There is no evidence that the POP has any effect either on the risk of breast cancer or benign breast problems. This means that, although there is no suggestion of it causing breast cancer, it does not appear to offer any of the protective effect that the COC gives against benign cysts and fibroadenomas either.

INJECTABLE PROGESTOGENS

The use of progestogen injections as a means of contraception was introduced in the 1960s. They are, however, quite unlike the combined and the progestogen-only pills.

The best known is Depo-Provera, a highly effective method of contraception given by an injection that gives contraceptive cover for 12 weeks. In the early 1980s it received a great deal of adverse publicity because some studies showed that beagle bitches given enormous doses were more likely to develop breast cancer. These studies highlighted the problems of extrapolating the results of experiments in animals to human beings, as it was later shown that beagles are prone to developing breast cancer anyhow, with or without Depo-Provera. Unfortunately, although much space was given to the original story, little was devoted to its later refutation. It should be stressed that there is no evidence to support an increased risk of breast cancer in women due to these progestogens.

HORMONE REPLACEMENT THERAPY

Since hormone replacement therapy (HRT) is given to women who are usually over 45, there has been much speculation as to whether it might influence the development of breast cancer, bearing in mind that women over 50 are in the highest risk group by virtue of their age.

Research on the relation between HRT use and breast cancer has given inconsistent results. Some studies do seem to suggest a small increase in risk if a woman had taken HRT for more than 10 years, but other studies show different findings. Obviously research is continuing and hopefully a clearer picture will soon emerge. For the present the significant benefits of HRT for some women outweigh this possible risk.

8

WHAT PLASTIC SURGERY CAN OFFER AND WHO SHOULD CONSIDER IT

Partly as a result of the vagaries of the fashion industry, few women are completely happy with every aspect of their appearance. This dissatisfaction often manifests itself in concern about the breasts – an important part of a woman's body image. She might think they are too small, in which case she may feel she lacks femininity; if she thinks they are too large she may be embarrassed by them. Sometimes there is a considerable difference in size between the two breasts.

People's assessment of what is the 'right' size and shape varies considerably, and some women are genuinely distressed by the size and shape of their breasts. They may feel inadequate or inhibited socially and sexually by their appearance. Such women may be helped a great deal by plastic surgery, and are usually happy with the results.

However, there is another group of women who request plastic surgery but who are seldom happy with the result, or who will then go on to find another feature of their body unattractive. These women are looking for an answer to a problem in their lives which may affect their self-esteem, but which actually has nothing to do with their figure. For example, a woman whose husband has been unfaithful may ask for plastic surgery, feeling herself to be unattractive. The surgery may change her appearance, but will not change the situation.

PRIOR CONSIDERATIONS

Therefore, before any woman decides to have plastic surgery of any kind, she should ask herself whether it is really her appearance alone that she wishes to change, or whether it is an excuse to avoid a more painful issue. Plastic surgery, like any surgery, can be painful, can leave scars, and can produce complications. In addition, since it is difficult to obtain on the NHS, it may involve considerable expense.

So, whenever you go to a plastic surgeon you will, or should, find that he or she will spend some time discussing with you why you want the operation. He or she will want to be sure that you are fully informed of the risks and benefits of any procedure, so that you will not be disappointed afterwards. A visit to a counsellor may even be suggested, if it is felt you need to discuss things more fully. Try not to be so dazzled by the possible results that you take no note of the possible complications; failure to do this can lead to disappointment later.

You also need to bear in mind that sweeping changes to your figure are not usually possible, and that what you think looks ideal on someone else may not be sensible for you. Again, these are aspects which you should discuss fully beforehand.

BREAST AUGMENTATION

This is the commonest plastic surgical operation on the breast. Silicone gel implants (prostheses) are the most widely used nowadays. They come in different shapes and sizes, so the end result can be tailored to suit each individual woman. Inflatable implants are sometimes used, but, as you can imagine, they have a tendency to deflate, which results in the need for a second operation.

There are several different ways of performing the breast augmentation operation, all of which have advantages and disadvantages. Your surgeon will undoubtedly have a preference, and you are best guided by him. (Apart from anything else, he is likely to be better at his preferred technique than any of the others!) It does not even necessarily have to be done using a general anaesthetic; a local anaesthetic and some Valium to relax you may be enough.

The incision, and therefore the scar, can be made in one of three different places. The most popular technique uses the low breast incision. The armpit incision looks better, but has been found to have more technical difficulties. Wherever the incision, the operation essentially involves introducing an implant into a space created either just above or below the main breast muscle, the pectoralis major. A small suction drain is usually inserted, and the operation usually results in two days in hospital.

Possible problems with breast augmentation
In about 20 per cent of women the body reacts to the silicon implant and makes a fibrous capsule around it. This has a tendency to contract and pull the soft breast-shaped implant into a tense round ball. It has been found that daily massage of the implant during the first few months helps to prevent this happening, so you will be shown how to do this. A technique known as popping can often relieve the problem; under a light anaesthetic the surgeon squeezes the breast until a popping sound is heard, as the capsule is dispersed and the implant is freed. If this fails, the fibrous capsule can be excised and a larger pocket made for the prosthesis.

The other main problem is loss of sensation around the nipple. The degree varies from woman to woman, but may be a source of disappointment if you are not prepared for the possibility. Other less common complications that can occur are:

• Bleeding into the wound in the first few days, usually dealt with by the suction drain.
• Infection, which usually requires removal of the prosthesis.
• Shifting of the prosthesis.
• And, very rarely, rupture of the prosthesis under the skin.

BREAST REDUCTION

Excessively large breasts can cause great embarrassment, as well as physical problems. The weight tends to cause poor posture and therefore backache. Many sporting activities, such as running or riding, are extremely uncomfortable, and some women feel too embarrassed even to wear a swimsuit. Intertrigo (fungal skin infection, see pages 33–4) can produce red infected skin in the moist areas under the breast, where it presses on the chest wall. Clothes are difficult to buy, and tend to be unfashionable, as fashion mainly caters for the slim figure. These handicaps all have to be weighed against the disadvantages of surgery, which leaves quite noticeable scars, but it is a reflection of the misery of large breasts that many women request the operation and are very pleased with the results.

The cause of disproportionately large breasts is not known – there is no obvious hormonal imbalance. Naturally, a woman who is considerably overweight is likely to have large breasts, but in those who are otherwise slim, losing weight does not seem to help a great deal.

Breast reduction is a more complicated procedure than augmentation, and leaves more obvious scars. In addition, nipple sensation is often reduced, and breastfeeding is no longer possible. Any woman considering it needs to be fully aware of the implications before she makes a decision.

There are several techniques in use. The basic idea is to remove areas of the breast symmetrically, preserving an acceptable shape. The nipple and areola are moved in order to maintain a normal appearance after the size of the breast has been changed. It is this removal and replacement of the nipple which causes the loss of sensation and of the ability to breastfeed, since the nerve endings to the nipple, and the milk ducts, have to be cut during the procedure. In addition, after the operation the woman is left with scars.

This operation is performed under a general anaesthetic, and usually involves a hospital stay of about four days. It takes about four weeks to feel fully recovered from the operation, and a supportive bra has to be worn day and night for six weeks.

Possible problems with breast reduction
The scars, loss of nipple sensation and the inability to breastfeed are inevitable consequences of this operation. Sometimes the scars become wider and more conspicuous if the blood supply to part of the breast tissue fails, or the incision does not heal well, and occasionally a skin graft is needed. If the blood supply to part of the breast tissue fails, tender lumpy areas are formed which usually soften after a few months. About half of the women who undergo this operation are likely

to have at least one of these problems. Nothing can be done about the loss of nipple sensation, but the scars can be removed surgically in the hope that the second ones will be better.

Another feature of the operation is the tendency for the breast to 'droop' with time. This can be corrected by another operation described in the next section. There is also little guarantee that the breast will be cosmetically 'perfect' – something which depends on many factors, including the expertise of the surgeon. Despite all these problems, the majority of women who choose to have this operation are pleased with the result.

'LIFTING' OF THE BREASTS (MASTOPEXY)

Breasts may sag with age or after pregnancy, as a result of gravity pulling downwards on the suspensory ligaments and the skin.

The operation of mastopexy only involves removing the skin and none of the breast tissue. The nipple and areola are moved, but are not detached from the underlying breast tissue, so nipple sensation is less affected than in breast reduction, and breastfeeding is still possible afterwards. It does leave scars, in the same position as in breast reduction, but they are shorter. Stretch marks in the lower part of the breast can be removed, but those in the skin over the upper part cannot.

Sometimes, if the breasts are also small, an implant is put in at the same time. This helps to maintain the shape better, but brings with it the complications of implants mentioned earlier in the chapter.

As after breast reduction, a bra must be worn day and night for six weeks.

BREAST RECONSTRUCTION AFTER MASTECTOMY

Breast reconstruction can be done after simple or radical mastectomy and, while it cannot replace a breast, it can produce a breast shape that fills the bra cup in the same way as the other breast, restoring a sense of balance, comfort and wholeness. It is also possible to construct a nipple that looks the same as the other side. This allows you to go swimming and play tennis, for example, without worries that an external prosthesis is going to slip, and removes the problem of the skin getting sweaty and uncomfortable under a silicon gel prosthesis in the bra cup.

The operation can be done at the time of the mastectomy or at any time thereafter – there is no time limit. However, the operation is not suitable for every patient who has had a mastectomy, and not all women want it. For example, those who have advanced breast cancer are not good candidates, and a number of other women prefer not to have any more operations involving painful reminders of what they have been through. The trend nowadays is towards doing less surgery, rather than more; furthermore fewer mastectomies are being performed. There is also the worry that the operation might mask recurrence of breast cancer until it is too advanced to treat easily. Nevertheless, most women who have their breast reconstructed are very pleased with the result.

What is involved?
There are a variety of different techniques for reconstructing a breast. Occasionally, if the skin is loose enough around the scar, all that is done is to insert a silicone prosthesis under the pectoralis muscle. However this is rarely possible, usually because the skin is too tight across the chest wall to allow satisfactory expansion, and without more tissue to bulk out the reconstructed breast it will still not match the other side well.

The usual procedure, therefore, is to use a myocutaneous flap – a flap of still-attached living healthy tissue composed of muscle and skin. The muscle is there partly to add tissue bulk and partly because the blood supply to the skin comes through the underlying muscle; if the skin is separated from the underlying muscle, it loses its blood supply. The muscle that can usually be most easily spared is the latissimus dorsi muscle from the back. Part of this muscle is removed, leaving almost no detectable weakness. Then, together with an ellipse of overlying fat and skin, it is brought round to the front, underneath the skin that runs down the side of the chest. All the while, this section of muscle, fat and skin is still attached at the top end, at the shoulder, so it remains healthy, with a good blood supply.

The original mastectomy scar is then opened and each side of this ellipse of skin is stitched to each side of the mastectomy scar, re-expanding it, with the associated bulk of muscle and fat immediately underneath. Usually a silicone prosthesis is needed in addition, so that by choosing the size and shape of the prosthesis the new breast shape can be increased as wanted.

Sometimes a myocutaneous flap is taken from the abdomen instead, particularly in a woman who is overweight. This can reduce the abdominal fat at the same time, but does tend to weaken the abdominal muscles slightly.

A nipple and areola can also be reconstructed, but this is usually done at a later operation. The areola skin is usually taken as a free graft from the skin of the thigh or the labia of the vulva because this is found to give the best colour match to the other areola. The nipple itself is usually fashioned by taking part of the opposite nipple, making two nipples that match closely, although the new nipple will not have any sensation.

Problems with breast reconstruction
From reading this description you will see what a major operation breast reconstruction is, and of course such an operation can have complications. For example, when the bra is removed the new breast is often firmer than the other side so the two breasts rarely match completely, the new one being better supported. This is partly as intended, because the aim is to make a shape that matches when a bra is being worn. One technique that can be used to make the two breasts match better is to carry out a reduction mammoplasty or a mastopexy on the other breast.

The two elliptical scars that cross the new breast are also inevitable, and in addition there will be a straight scar across the back. The ellipse of new skin may even have a very slightly different colour to the rest of the skin, although this can be masked easily.

Complications that can occur include infection leading to increased scarring, and breakdown of skin from necrosis if the blood supply is inadequate. Scarring around the silicone implant can also occur as a result of the body's reaction; this leads to a tense tennis-ball shape, but may be minimised by daily massage or by 'popping' (disrupting of the capsule by the surgeon under sedation) or by surgery under anaesthetic.

HOW TO GO ABOUT OBTAINING PLASTIC SURGERY

How do you find a good and reputable plastic surgeon? This is a very difficult question, as there is a shortage of such surgeons in the National Health Service in Britain. The field is therefore open for those who are more interested in your money than your welfare. This is not to say that a surgeon in private practice will not be good. Indeed, the opposite may well be the case; if he spends all his time on cosmetic surgery, he may well be superb. But how can you, a non-medical person, discriminate?

In the case of reconstructive surgery you are at an advantage, since you are already under the care of a consultant surgeon who specialises in breast disease. He is therefore likely to know of a good surgeon, whose results he has seen and in whom he has confidence. It is quite likely that he will know of both NHS and private practice surgeons, and will be able to discuss the advantages and disadvantages of each with you.

If you are seeking purely cosmetic surgery, however, the situation is slightly more difficult. The first step is to see your doctor. He or she may know of a good plastic surgeon, in which case your problem is solved. If this is not the case, ask your doctor to write to:

The Honorary Secretary
British Association of Plastic Surgeons
35 Lincoln's Inn Fields, London WC2

This association consists of reputable surgeons who hold an NHS post, although they may also do private work. They will provide your doctor with a list of members who are primarily experts in reconstructive surgery but who may also do more cosmetic operations. There is a second association, the Association of Aesthetic Plastic Surgeons, whose members specialise in the more cosmetic aspects of plastic surgery. Once again, your doctor can obtain a list by writing to the same address.

Do not contact these organisations yourself, as you will be disappointed; they are only allowed to give information about their members to a doctor. However, your GP or clinic doctor is unlikely to refuse your request for information, especially if you are able to provide the necessary address. Indeed, they should be reassured that you will be in good hands as a result of their efforts.

71

9

GENERAL INFORMATION ABOUT BREAST CANCER

The word cancer is always frightening. It refers to a disease that can start without warning or apparent cause, and in certain cases no cure is possible, in spite of all the recent medical developments. Because of this the word 'cancer' is often interpreted as 'incurable', whereas in reality it can often be completely and permanently cured, most particularly if it is found in its early stages.

The word 'cancer' is in fact Latin for 'crab', and this will be familiar to you if you know the signs of the zodiac. The word is applied to this disease presumably because of the 'claws' that it puts out into the surrounding tissues.

WHAT IS CANCER?

A cancer is one type of tumour or growth. These words may sound nearly as unpleasant as cancer, but there are completely benign harmless tumours as well as malignant ones. A fatty lump called a lipoma is a common example of a harmless benign tumour, and benign breast tumours are common. A benign tumour is a collection of cells that just gets bigger; it may squeeze the surrounding tissue, but it does not otherwise damage it.

However, a tumour may be malignant. This means that, if they are allowed to, the abnormal-looking cells that it contains can spread within the body, start off other tumours and go on to destroy normal tissue. And it is these malignant tumours that have the term cancer applied to them. Cancers can be of different types – the medical terms carcinoma, sarcoma and

72

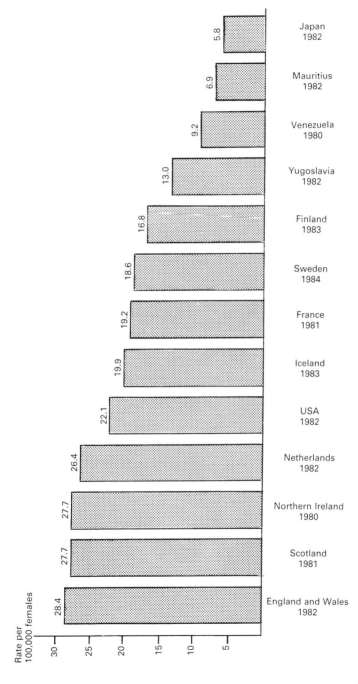

Rate per 100,000 females

Mortality rates from breast cancer for women of the same age in various countries.

Country	Year	Rate
Japan	1982	5.8
Mauritius	1982	6.9
Venezuela	1980	9.2
Yugoslavia	1982	13.0
Finland	1983	16.8
Sweden	1984	18.6
France	1981	19.2
Iceland	1983	19.9
USA	1982	22.1
Netherlands	1982	26.4
Northern Ireland	1980	27.7
Scotland	1981	27.7
England and Wales	1982	28.4

73

lymphoma are examples of different types of cancer, with carcinoma being the commonest cancer.

Carcinoma can start in most organs of the body. In women the commonest starting place for cancer is the breast – one woman in 14 in the UK will develop breast cancer, with a total of 25,000 new breast cancers developing every year in the UK. And this number is slowly rising.

WHO IS MOST LIKELY TO GET BREAST CANCER?

Age
The average age of those developing breast cancer is 55 years. However, the age range is wide and breast cancer can occasionally occur in teenagers or 90 year olds.

Menarche and menopause
Breast cancer is commoner in those who have an earlier first period (the menarche), at 12 years of age or less. It is also commoner in those women who have a late menopause.

Number of children
Breast cancer is slightly commoner in women who have had no children. For a long time it was thought that the more children a woman had, the greater her protection against breast cancer. However it has now been shown that the important factor is the age at which she has her first child – the earlier a woman has her first child, the lower her risk of breast cancer. If a woman has her first child when she is young, there is a greater chance of her having more children; this is why it appeared that large numbers of children were a protective factor. Only full-term pregnancies appear to be protective – miscarriages or abortions have no effect.

The critical age for this protective effect of pregnancy seems to be for a woman to have her first child before the age of 32. However there is even greater protection if this first child is born before a woman is 25 years old.

Breastfeeding
Breast cancer is slightly commoner in those women who have not breastfed. It seems, however, that breastfeeding has to

74

continue for some years rather than for a few months if this is to provide a significant protective effect.

Family history
A woman who has a sister or a mother with breast cancer has a two-fold increased risk of getting a breast cancer herself. The age at which her relative had breast cancer is important: if the relative's cancer developed after the age of 50 then the risk is only increased from the average of one in 14 to one in eight; but if she was less than 50 then the risk to the woman is about one in four. If it was her aunt or grandmother who was affected by breast cancer, then she is at a slightly increased risk as well, and if more than one relative had breast cancer the risk is increased even further. Furthermore, in those women who do have a relevant family history, the age of onset tends to be younger with each successive generation; if you get past this period of risk without developing cancer, then as you get older the increased risk disappears.

All this only applies if it was breast cancer that the relative had; it does not apply if there was any other type of cancer in the family.

Different countries
There is a considerable variation in risk in different countries. Women in Japan have the lowest risk and the UK has the highest – higher even than the rest of Europe and North America. However, the incidence of breast cancer is increasing everywhere, most particularly so in Japan.

Chronic liver disease and alcohol
Women who have severe chronic liver disease have an increased incidence of breast cancer. Additionally, women who regularly drink more than nine measures of spirits, glasses of wine or pints of beer per week have nearly double the risk of breast cancer, although this may be due to the liver problems that occur. Smaller amounts of alcohol that cause no damage to the liver appear to have no influence on the development of breast cancer.

Obesity
Women who are considerably overweight are more likely to get breast cancer.

Social class
Breast cancer is more common in the higher social classes.

Radiation
Women who have been exposed to excessive radiation are more likely to develop breast cancer. Studies on the survivors of the atomic bombs dropped on Hiroshima and Nagasaki showed that women who were girls of 10 years or less when the bombs were dropped had an increased chance of developing breast cancer, with the risk being proportional to the amount of radiation they had received. The cancers usually developed about 20 years after the exposure to radiation.

Studies of girls with tuberculosis showed that more of them developed breast cancers than expected in later life, and there seems no doubt that this was due to all the chest X-rays they received in childhood. The earliest mammograms gave relatively high doses of radiation, and were associated with an increased incidence of subsequent breast cancer which seems to be due to the radiation; it was as a result of these findings that the radiation dosage given in mammograms has been drastically reduced.

The cancers produced by radiation are identical to other cancers.

Previous breast cancer
A breast cancer occurring in one breast makes it more likely that a second new cancer will develop in the other breast. A woman who has already had a breast cancer therefore has an increased chance of getting a cancer in the other breast. This is not spread from the first cancer but is a new one starting.

It is important to realise that these associations have no bearing on deciding whether the breast lump in an individual woman is a cancer or not. Because you may fall into one or more of these risk categories, you cannot assume that merely because you have a breast lump it will necessarily be a cancer – being in a risk category plays no part in helping doctors decide if a lump is a cancer.

WHAT CAUSES BREAST CANCER?

We now understand a lot about how cancers start, but sadly there are still large gaps in this knowledge. It seems that most cells have the potential within them to keep on dividing and turn into a cancer, but this is usually kept in check. This malignant potential, which is rather like a time bomb, occurs because somewhere on the chromosome (the inherited genetic material in each cell that controls its activity) there is an area (a gene) called an oncogene (meaning a tumour-causing gene). In normal cells these oncogenes seem to have no useful function, and lie dormant and inactive. In malignant cells, however, they become active, because another gene which was acting as a controlling 'brake' gets damaged because the oncogene moves to a different part of the chromosome where it is easier for it to become active, or because an extra oncogene gets into the cell.

Fortunately, even if a cell does go wrong, the body's defence system normally spots it and destroys it. So cancer only develops when a cell with an active oncogene has escaped the body's defences and has got established.

It seems that many physical and chemical agents can damage the controlling 'brake' on the oncogene. We have already seen that radiation increases the risk of a cancer developing, probably by causing direct damage to the genes. However the vast majority of women who develop breast cancer do not receive significant amounts of such radiation; the few chest X-rays and mammograms they may have will have been little different to the normal background radiation.

There must therefore be other factors to explain why they have developed breast cancer. Of course it may be that the development of breast cancer simply occurs at random, or it may be that there is more than one factor that sets it off. Some of the reasons that have been considered are as follows.

Stress

It used to be thought that stress caused cancer. Sir James Paget wrote in 1870: 'The cases are so frequent in which deep anxiety, deferred hope and disappointment are quickly followed by the growth and increase of cancer that we can hardly doubt that mental depression is a weighty additive to the other influences favouring the development of the cancerous constitution.' Well nowadays we do doubt it!

There followed many reports of people who had a bereavement in the family, became depressed and then developed cancer themselves. It seemed as though there might be some truth in this suggestion, so two large studies were set up of people who had had a recent bereavement, to see if they were more likely to develop cancer. One looked at a 1 per cent sample of the England and Wales population and the other, in 1983, looked at all women in Denmark under the age of 70, and both these studies showed no evidence of a link between stress or particular personality types and the development of cancer.

Trauma
Knocks and bangs on the breast have never been found to cause any breast cancer. Often women think a cancer started with a knock, but this is usually because they went to rub themselves after a knock and their attention was then drawn to the lump.

Animal fats
You will remember from page 73 that there is a considerable variation in the risk of breast cancer in different countries. The explanation for this differing incidence that fits best is that it is caused by different intakes of animal fats – breast cancer incidence in different countries closely matches animal fat intake.

Furthermore, we know that the different incidences are not due to genetic differences. Studies of Japanese women (there is a low incidence of breast cancer in Japan) who moved to the United States of America, where there is high incidence, found that their children had a greater chance of getting breast cancer, and their grandchildren had the same chance as other Americans, presumably because of the new eating habits they had acquired in their new home.

The fast-rising incidence of breast cancer in Japan is assumed to be due to the rapid increase in animal-fat intake occurring in that country.

Hormones
There is some evidence that the naturally produced hormones oestrogen and prolactin found circulating in the body may play an important part in causing breast cancers to grow. For example, if a breast cancer develops during breastfeeding, when there is a high level of both these hormones in the blood, then it grows very rapidly.

Perhaps these circulating naturally produced hormones make the right climate for breast cancer to start. This would explain why there is a greater chance of getting a breast cancer when the periods start earlier or there is a late menopause, both allowing a longer time for stimulation of the breast by these hormones. This could also explain the relationship between breast cancer and liver disease; the liver makes a protein that binds (effectively 'locks up') oestrogen, so if the liver is damaged less oestrogen will be bound and more of it will be left to stimulate the breast.

When artificial oestrogens are given (for example in the pill), they stop the production of natural oestrogen in the body. It is still unclear whether or not these artificial oestrogens have any effect; this is discussed at some length in Chapter 7.

Viruses

For many years it has been known that viruses can cause breast cancer in mice and that mice can pass this virus on to their young in their breastmilk. The scientist who discovered this, Dr Bitner, thought he found the same virus particles in human cancers as long ago as 1936. It was also found that serum (blood fluid) from women with breast cancer can protect mice from being infected with the mouse breast-cancer virus and this raised great hopes of developing a serum which would do the same for humans.

However, in spite of many years of research, no such anti-cancer serum has been found. Indeed, there is still no definite evidence that human breast cancer is actually started by a virus – it may be that viruses just get into the cancer after it develops. This research is still going on; one study was reported in the medical journal the *Lancet* in 1988 which found evidence that viruses called retroviruses are more commonly found in the blood of women with breast cancer.

CAN I CATCH IT?

No contact, however close, whether by touching, doing dressings, or contact with blood, can transmit breast cancer from one person to another. There is also no evidence of transmission of any breast-cancer-causing effect from mother to baby by breastfeeding.

79

CAN I PREVENT IT?

So many of even the known risk factors for breast cancer are outside our control; you cannot, for instance, choose to have a mother who never gets breast cancer and you cannot decide the age of your first period. Since there is so little that can be done to prevent breast cancer developing, by far the most important measure you can therefore take is to concentrate on early diagnosis by self-examination and mammography screening. If the diagnosis can be made early, then the chance of curing it is much higher.

However there are a few things that you can do to reduce the risks. It may well help if you breastfeed your baby, if you avoid becoming overweight and if you keep your alcohol consumption down to moderate levels. And doctors need to be careful not to carry out any unnecessary X-rays on girls.

With all the evidence about animal fats given above you would think that keeping to a low animal-fat diet would help. The United States National Cancer Institute is considering funding a large study in America to reduce fat intake and see if it results in a reduced breast-cancer incidence, although so far there is no evidence that changing to a low animal-fat diet will decrease the chance of getting a breast cancer. However, in the same way as it is radiation in childhood that is important in causing cancer, so it may be that this is the critical time for other causes; if low animal-fat diets are started early in life they could well show an effect on reducing the risk of breast cancer. So, although there is good reason to suppose that cutting down on animal fats ought to help, making changes to your diet now may be too late; what we should perhaps be doing is encouraging our children to improve their diets. Supplementing diets with essential fatty acids might help, although as yet there is no evidence.

There are other measures that could be considered for women who are at high risk, perhaps because of a family history of breast cancer. Reducing ovarian activity would be a help. It would not be practical to do this by removing the ovaries after childbearing, because there is an increased risk of developing cardiovascular disease and osteoporosis, to say nothing of the emotional and psychological effects, although this would reduce the chance of getting a breast cancer. There are reasons to think that giving the anti-oestrogen drug tamoxifen to high-risk women would help, though, and a trial is planned. However such treatment would have to be started early because breast cancers start many years before they are clinically apparent. A minor worry is that if tumours did still develop, they might then be insensitive to this useful drug.

Finally, some women at particularly high risk have been treated by bilateral subcutaneous mastectomy before a cancer has developed, removing all the breast tissue but preserving the skin of the breast and the nipple, so that a prosthesis that matches the removed breast as closely as possible can be slipped into the resulting space. This operation has most often been carried out in America, and most often on one side only, after a cancer has developed on the other side. This is only rarely the best solution to the problem of being in a high-risk group; relying on screening is usually best.

WHERE DOES IT START IN THE BREAST?

It is thought that breast cancer starts in a single cell in the breast; cancers that seem to have started in several cells in different parts of the breast are known, but are very uncommon. The single cancer cell divides to make two cancer cells, these divide to make four cancer cells, then eight, then sixteen, and so on, until a recognisable lump of cells is formed. Along the way bits of the cancer may spread to other parts of the breast, or travel in the lymph system or bloodstream outside the breast.

The initial cancer cell that starts the process off may occur in any part of the breast – in a lobule or a duct, for example. This gives rise to slightly different characteristics to cancers, so that we can recognise a lobular cancer or a ductal cancer. Occasionally breast cancer seems to start at the nipple, producing a red itchiness of the nipple known as Paget's disease. In fact these malignant cancer cells originate in the ducts just underneath the nipple and migrate up the ducts to the nipple – the nipple itself never seems to be the source of a cancer.

WHAT DOES CANCER LOOK LIKE?

Cancer produces a very firm greyish-white tissue, with irregular margins where it is invading the normal surrounding tissue. It often feels gritty when cut because of the flecks of hard calcium in it (it is these calcium deposits that make the small white dots on a mammogram). The tumour usually pulls on the fibrous strands that run through the breast, and it is this action that leads to the dimpling of the overlying skin, distortion of the contour of the breast or retraction of the nipple.

Under the microscope many different appearances can be identified, and these appearances provide a whole lot more technical terms that doctors use when categorising a particular patient's carcinoma. These categories are important because the different types develop in different ways, making it sometimes possible to predict future developments from the appearances seen.

Any tumour that is removed is always sent to a pathologist, who provides a detailed report of its naked-eye and microscopic appearances (this usually takes several days). Words like lobular, ductal, medullary, scirrhous and *in situ* are all used; for instance *in situ* is the earliest stage in the development of a cancer, before it has started to spread within the breast and become invasive – while it is *in situ* it is completely curable. The pathologist's report also uses the term grade, which means how closely the cells are arranged like the ducts and tubules of normal breast tissue; the cancer is called well differentiated if it is similar in arrangement to normal breast tissue (this will be a less aggressive cancer), and poorly differentiated if it just consists of sheets of malignant cells (which will tend to spread earlier and be more resistant to treatment).

When the pathologist looks at the tumour under the microscope he or she will also often be able to see signs of the body's defence mechanisms attacking the tumour. These defences can kill malignant cells, particularly small clumps and isolated cells, but unfortunately are less effective when attacking a solid mass of tumour.

HOW QUICKLY DOES CANCER GROW?

The growth rate of a cancer varies in different instances. It can be slowed or even stopped by changes in hormone levels, and by the body's defences as well as by anti-cancer medicines and radiotherapy.

An average growth rate is for the cells in a tumour to divide once every 100 days, and from that it can be calculated that it takes a cancer about seven-and-a-half years to grow from a single cell to a pea-sized lump about a centimetre (half an inch) across – the size when it should be just big enough to feel. It has to be admitted that this knowledge about cancer growth is not often publicised by doctors; it is a worrying thought for a woman that a pea-size tumour has been growing in her breast for over seven years, and once this fact is realised it can make it difficult to encourage her to seek medical advice quickly.

However there is a very good reason for seeking rapid treatment. The cancer cells have a constant 'doubling time', so each 100 days there will be first two cells, then four cells, then eight cells, 16 cells, etc. It therefore remains a microscopic size for a long time; after 20 doubling times (and that will take five years) it will have only reached a millimetre across – still hardly visible to the naked eye. However it then takes only another ten cell divisions (another two-and-a-half years) to grow to a centimetre across. And from then on it seems as though there is an enormous acceleration in the perceived growth rate, even though it is still produced as before by each cell dividing every 100 days.

A very rare situation, and one in which breast cancer appears to grow more rapidly than usual, is when it develops in a woman who is breastfeeding. This may be because of the increased bloodflow to the breast at this time and the increase in circulating hormones, both of which may stimulate the tumour.

Tamoxifen is a drug which acts as an anti-oestrogen, and has been shown to slow down the growth rate of breast cancers.

HOW DOES CANCER SPREAD?

A cancer starts to spread by pushing out in between surrounding normal cells and then goes on to destroy them. After a while it gets into the lymphatic channels, and the cancer cells can then be transported in the lymph. Once they get into the lymphatic system they will be transported to the lymph nodes, usually starting with the nodes in the axilla (armpit). Here they may be destroyed by the body's defences. However, if these defences are beaten the cancer cells will start to grow in the lymph node, and if unchecked they may get into the bloodstream and can then spread anywhere in the body. They do have certain places where they prefer to grow, however, principally the bones, the lungs and the liver.

The clump of malignant cells where the cancer starts in the breast is called the primary tumour. When it spreads and starts growing elsewhere in the body, these new clumps of tumour cells are called secondaries or metastases.

At what stage does a cancer start to spread?

It used to be thought that breast cancers spread in an orderly fashion, first locally, then to the lymph nodes and finally beyond the nodes into the bloodstream. We now know that individual cells break off into the bloodstream at an early stage. However, whereas the body's defences are not good at dealing with a solid mass of tumour cells, they are good at destroying individual cancer cells.

We not know how soon these cancer cells start to spread away from a breast cancer. It may well vary with different cancers, but it is probable that by the time most cancers are clinically detected some malignant cells will have been spread from them, although they may not necessarily have survived.

HOW DOES BREAST CANCER KILL?

Cancer usually causes death by malnutrition. The cancer produces toxins (poisons) which get into the bloodstream and have the effect of taking away the appetite. This effect builds up as the tumour grows, and only really becomes apparent when the tumour is advanced.

This does not mean that loss of appetite is any help in diagnosis of breast cancer; it is far more likely to be due to anxiety in the early stages. However, late in the course of the disease loss of appetite leads to weight loss and weakness. In this weak state awareness of what is going on is often gradually reduced. Reduced resistance to infection is another consequence of the reduced nutritional intake, and subsequent infection in the chest is often the final straw that is too much for the body to cope with.

Other effects on the body from the tumour may be distressing, but they are not usually the cause of death. Sometimes the tumour may press on the chest wall and make an unsightly ulcer, although an important aim of treatment is to prevent this happening. Secondary tumours may cause pain and fractures in bones, or fluid on the lung, or may interfere with the working of the liver and cause jaundice.

10

TREATMENT OF BREAST CANCER

Hearing a diagnosis of breast cancer is frightening. You have an unknown and perhaps threatening course of treatment ahead of you, and there are so many confusing questions. Will it involve mutilating surgery? Will it be painful? Is the doctor sure of the diagnosis anyway? Perhaps it is all a mistake. Of course you want to get it dealt with as quickly as possible, but are you being guided on the best course? Are you in the best hands? Are you able to put all your trust in the specialist who is advising you? Is it all worthwhile anyway? Perhaps there would be alternative gentler treatments than surgery.

You will probably be told the diagnosis by the consultant surgeon who has done a biopsy, and until that biopsy result is obtained you can never be certain of the diagnosis. The consultant will then explain what other tests are needed and what treatments are recommended for you.

THE DIFFERENT TREATMENT OPTIONS

It is at this point that you are faced with the realisation that there is not just one standard treatment for breast cancer that everyone agrees is best, but instead a whole range of treatments. Individual surgeons favour different operations, and each medical specialist, radiotherapist and oncologist will weigh up problems differently and recommend slightly different solutions.

Many women in fact want to consider all the treatment options that are available, and doctors often underestimate the amount of information their patients want. Some specialists

86

are not very forthcoming about the different treatment options because they realise that for a woman to be faced with a range of options at this time can be frightening and confusing. And some women in fact prefer to go to a specialist they can trust and then accept the advice they get – choices can create more anxiety at this very worrying time. Furthermore, if the decision is left to the patient, without the specialist making a strong personal recommendation, it can often make the specialist appear indecisive. Perhaps the best approach is for the specialist to explain the options and then to make recommendations.

You should therefore be offered every opportunity to ask questions and discuss the plan of treatment. And even if you are not given such opportunities, do not be shy – just ask. There may of course be so many questions you want to ask that you forget some, in which case it is often a good idea to make a list of the important ones. If you go in to see the specialist with a relative or close friend the extra support may help you to go calmly through all the questions you want answered. This book of course assumes that you want to be well informed about the problems and their solutions. In that way you can become a 'member of the team', working with your specialists to decide what is the right treatment for you. This in turn gives you a degree of control in what is going on and, at the same time, greater trust in those advising you. If you are sure you are getting the best treatment you will get through this difficult time more easily.

In the past radical mastectomy was the preferred operation, in the hope that the more thoroughly the tumour and surrounding tissue was removed the higher would be the cure rate. This led to anxiety in the woman's mind about what was often perceived as disfiguring treatment (mastectomy), these worries sometimes being as great as those about the disease itself. Furthermore, at that time biopsies had to be done under a general anaesthetic, and general anaesthetics then were less safe than they are today. It was therefore considered important to remove the cancer completely at the same time as the biopsy was taken, so the tumour had less chance to spread, and only one anaesthetic was given. The consequence of this was that women went to the operation not actually knowing if it was going to involve a mastectomy or not.

Fortunately a lot has happened in recent years to make a

vast improvement to breast cancer treatment. Evidence has come from careful clinical trials that simpler operations can give just as good a cure rate. Biopsies can now be done very simply and easily with a needle, and without a general anaesthetic. And there is not the same urgency to get a tumour removed before a single cell has escaped – it is known now that cells are escaping from tumours into the bloodstream all the time. Although this sounds even more worrying, it actually means that the body's defences are much better at killing off stray cancer cells than was originally thought.

The earliest radical mastectomies (Halstedt mastectomies) involved removing the breast and the lymph nodes in the armpit (axilla), together with the pectoralis muscles that spread out over the chest wall. Later, modified radical mastectomies (Patey mastectomies) were introduced which also removed the breast, the axillary nodes and the deeper pectoralis minor muscle, but not the overlying and larger pectoralis major muscle, so the shoulder looked much more normal.

Now it is generally agreed that it is important to get the best cure rate with the least distorting and damaging operation. This means that for many women cures are obtained by a local excision (usually called lumpectomy) of a cancer, often through a small incision, the cancer being removed with only a small margin of normal tissue, leaving little distortion of the breast, especially if the cancer was small. If necessary, a separate incision in the armpit can be made, either to take out just one or two lymph nodes to see if they are involved or to clear them all away.

Equally good survival rates are obtained by this much more acceptable surgery, although there is a higher chance of local recurrence. The operation is therefore usually followed by radiotherapy to the breast, to try to kill any cancer cells left in the area. The final result is usually just a small scar on the breast and very little visible evidence of the treated cancer. The radiotherapy also needs to be given to the armpit unless the nodes have been cleared from there.

A further very new development is that it is sometimes considered safe to avoid radiotherapy completely for some patients and give them tamoxifen instead. Trials are underway to make sure this is as safe as giving radiotherapy. This removes worries about the possible long-term effects of radiotherapy, which can always be given later if necessary.

This does not mean that simple and radical mastectomies are not sometimes used. Mastectomy is still usually best for tumours that start in several different parts of the breast at the same time (called multifocal) or if the tumour is large and located in a central position in the breast. Removing just the lump alone would leave such a small distorted breast that mastectomy, possibly followed by reconstruction, is considered better. If a mastectomy is performed, radiotherapy is usually not given; for this reason, some women, particularly those over 60, actually prefer this option. Although there is no evidence that mastectomy gives longer survival, it does produce a smaller risk of local recurrence than local surgery.

If the cancer is locally advanced, involving skin or muscle, or if there are secondary tumours (metastases) in other parts of the body, then the treatment is usually radiotherapy with the addition of endocrine (hormone) therapy and sometimes chemotherapy.

In deciding which is the best treatment for an individual, her age, menopausal state, tumour size, local spread, lymph node involvement and metastases in other parts of the body all need to be taken into account, together with the woman's own views on the different treatments. Each treatment has advantages and disadvantages, often quite small ones, so it may come about that different specialists recommend different treatments. This is hardly likely to produce confidence in the patient. However it does not mean it is a good idea to shop around until you find someone who recommends the treatment you hoped would be recommended; such treatment may prove not to be the best for you.

DOUBTS ABOUT SURGERY

Many people worry that surgery will 'stir up' a tumour and encourage it to spring up elsewhere, either because the surgery causes malignant cells to be sent off around the body or perhaps because the body and its natural defences will be weakened by the operation. These worries may stem from hearing of someone whose tumour seemed to progress rapidly after surgery; if that is the case, the situation usually arose because they went to see their doctor at too late a stage, when the tumour had already spread extensively. There are sometimes worries that surgery is 'unnatural' compared to alternative treatments. Sometimes there are worries that full detailed scans should be done before operation; if the cancer has already spread it might make surgery unnecessary. Since it is known that the lymph nodes are part of the body's defences, it is a natural concern that if the operation is going to remove them then resistance might be reduced.

In the present state of our knowledge, there is no evidence that any more malignant cells get into the bloodstream during an operation than were doing so earlier; and once the tumour is out no more malignant cells can get into the bloodstream. Furthermore, the body contains a vast number of lymph nodes (there are about 200 in the neck alone) and removing a few nodes in the armpit produces no measurable reduction in the body's defences.

So, all the evidence suggests that the sooner the primary tumour is out of the body the better. If it is small and has not spread from the breast it will be permanently cured by surgery, and even if it has already spread it is still important to remove the primary tumour to stop further spread and at least to make sure that it does not progress any further in the breast.

TALKING TO YOUR SPECIALIST

It will most likely be a surgeon who has done the biopsy that gives the diagnosis and who will then be the person who explains to you that the result showed a cancer. After taking a full history and carrying out a thorough examination and probably a chest X-ray, some blood tests and possibly X-rays of your spine and pelvis, you will sit down together in the outpatient clinic to discuss what the position is and what the treatment should be. Do not think that surgeons only recommend surgical treatment. Not only do they treat many patients with non-surgical techniques but they also work closely with the rest of the team that will include a medical oncologist (a cancer specialist who uses medicines rather than surgery or radiotherapy to treat cancer), a radiotherapist and a nurse counsellor.

Ask all the questions you want to ask. Ask to look at the biopsy report if you want. It is good to be an active participant in deciding what treatment is best for you, so get the surgeon to explain fully what is recommended for you and why he or she does not recommend the other options.

You can decide on how long an interval you want before any operation that is proposed, but it certainly helps avoid future worries if you can agree on dates there and then. You may need some time to go and consider what you have heard and to discuss it more – an interval of a week or two will do no harm – but the operation is usually arranged as soon as possible to reduce the anxiety of waiting. You will have a lot to do in this time, making arrangements for home and work; you should try and give yourself time to meet friends, though, and do not isolate yourself.

In America the surgeon will tell you every complication that could possibly happen, which makes fairly worrying listening. In the UK you will be told about the likely complications, and any others that you ask about, but probably not about complications that only have a tiny chance of happening. For instance, there is roughly a one in 3,000 chance that a breast operation will be followed by a blood clot on the lung; because this is so unlikely it will most probably not be mentioned, unless you ask about it. American surgeons, of course, are more concerned about whether or not they are going to be sued if something goes wrong and they have not mentioned this possibility; it is for this reason that they mention every possible complication, rather than because it is really best for the patient. In the UK you can expect to be told of every complication or risk that is important or likely.

OPERATIONS

You will usually be admitted to hospital on the day before the operation if you are to have a general anaesthetic. If you will be having an operation under local anaesthetic, though, you will often be admitted on the same day as the operation. A junior member of the surgical team – a houseman or registrar – will then go through your history with you again and examine you. If it is a teaching hospital it is up to you if you want to see medical students and let them examine you, but remember that your consultant only got the expertise and experience that you are now grateful for by starting as a medical student.

Moreover you may find that talking to the medical students and to the nurses helps, not only to pass the time but also to pick up all sorts of practical information about the hospital and the operation. Another visit you will receive is from your anaesthetist, who will check on your fitness for the operation and tell you about the anaesthetic. There will also be further opportunities to talk to your surgeon and the rest of the team (registrar and house-surgeon, nurse counsellor and ward sister) about the proposed operation.

Of course nothing can be done to you in hospital without your consent, so there will be a consent form brought round for you to sign. Before you do sign it, though, you should be completely clear about what operation is being done, why that operation was decided upon, what is to be removed, where the scars will be, and what the appearance will be afterwards. The consent form will not specify who is going to do the operation; often, of course, it will be a team of two or even three people. If you want to know exactly who will do what, then just ask.

On the consent form there will be a clause that says you agree to 'anything else that may be necessary' or 'further or alternative measures', which can be a very confusing and worrying legal technicality. This might sound a rather open-ended clause; however, if, for instance, you have agreed to a lumpectomy it should be quite clear that that would *not* include consent to mastectomy. If you have any worries about what might be done, in addition to writing what operation you agree to you can also write on the consent form what you would not agree to, e.g. 'lumpectomy but not mastectomy'. In practice, though, if you have discussed the operation fully and clearly with your surgeon, so that you both agree on what is to be done, there should be no need for any such additions to the form or any worries about what will actually be done.

Before the operation you will have a shower or a bath. You may not have another opportunity to wash your hair for many days, so take the chance while it is there. Make sure family and friends know what number to ring to get information about you, and when they can visit. It is useful if one person agrees to let the rest of your family and friends know how you are so that the others do not have the problems of ringing through to the ward individually. You will have nothing to eat or drink for at least four hours before the operation, and if the operation is in the morning you will usually be asked to have nothing after midnight. Then about an hour before the operation the ward nurse will give you a 'pre-med', an intramuscular injection in your bottom that makes you sleepy and makes your mouth dry.

When you get to the anacsthetic room beside the theatre you will still be awake, but drowsy. There will be checks again in the anaesthetic room that you are the right person having the right operation and that you have had nothing to eat or drink before the operation, etc. Usually a mark will have been put on the skin beside the lump and this will be checked as well. The surgeon will come in to say hello and then the anaesthetist will give you an intravenous injection that lets you drift off to sleep in a few seconds.

Lumpectomy

This means that just the lump, and not the rest of the breast, is removed. It is sometimes called a 'local excision' and it can usually be done through a fairly small incision, although this depends on the size of the tumour and where it is in the breast. If possible the cut is made in the skin crease or around the areola to make it as inconspicuous as possible. The lump is removed, plus some surrounding tissue to get a clear margin, and this usually leaves little or no distortion of the contour of the breast. There may be a separate incision to remove the lymph nodes in the armpit (axilla).

You may have a small suction drain to suck out any blood that accumulates in the wound; this is removed when it is no longer draining. You will probably be able to leave the hospital between one and three days after the operation.

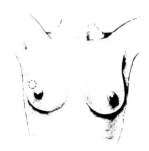

Lumpectomy.

93

Simple mastectomy

In this operation the whole of the breast is removed, including the nipple but not the lymph nodes in the armpit. The chest wall will be flat afterwards, almost certainly with a transverse scar, but the pectoralis muscle will be untouched. You will probably have a suction drain – a tube coming from near the scar, with an attached bottle – and will remain in hospital for about five days. Getting full shoulder movement back is usually easy.

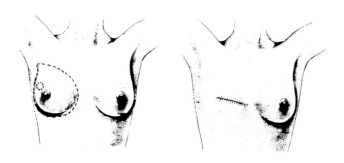

Simple mastectomy.

Radical mastectomy

The word 'radical' means that the nodes in the armpit are removed as well as the breast and, although nowadays the pectoralis major muscle is not removed, the little pectoralis minor muscle underneath is usually removed in order to get at

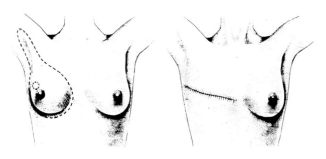

Radical mastectomy.

94

all the lymph nodes. However this does not produce any noticeable weakness in the shoulder. Nevertheless, because the lymphatic vessels are divided, there are usually two suction drains and these stay in until the body has made new channels to take away the lymph, after about seven days. In the majority of cases the scar will be transverse and will look almost the same as for a simple mastectomy.

After the operation
From the theatre you go to the recovery room for about half an hour and then back to the ward. There is not likely to be much pain, but you can ask for whatever painkillers you need. You will not need to stay in bed, and in fact will be encouraged to sit in a chair and walk, although at first when you stand you may feel a little dizzy – and you will need to remember to pick up any drainage bottles that are attached to your suction drain. The physiotherapist will visit you with exercises for your chest and legs, as well as the arm and shoulder on the side of the operation. There will also be some routine blood tests.

The wound needs to be kept dry for about six days. The drainage tubes pull out quite easily, and if there are stitches or clips to remove this is done after about a week, although nowadays you may have absorbable stitches underneath the skin.

If you have had a mastectomy then looking at the scar for the first time is always a difficult moment, probably better not delayed. You will be given a soft temporary prosthesis to put in the bra cup that you can use until the scar has healed. You may be visited by a nurse counsellor during this time.

It can take up to a week for the histology (study of cells) report to come through from the laboratory with details of the tumour that was removed, and when it does the surgeon will come and discuss it with you.

AT HOME

Often when you get home after such an operation, tiredness and depression flood over you as what has happened really sinks in. It is easier to cope well in hospital, where there is so much happening, with nurses and doctors bustling around, but at home you have more time on your own. It can be depressing realising how tired you get climbing stairs or going out for a walk. You are back in the real world and now you are on your own.

You do need some time on your own, but do not isolate yourself. Get family and friends to help with washing and cleaning. Do not worry that you find you need more sleep – have an afternoon nap. Your concentration and memory will seem to be affected, too, so that even reading a novel will be difficult. Eat as well as you can to regain your strength.

There are no hard and fast rules because everyone is different but you will know yourself how much you can do in terms of getting out for walks or to visit friends. Tiring yourself a little but not too much, and doing a little more each day, is a good plan to work to. You may think your tiredness is out of proportion to the healing that is taking place, but when the body has been injured it diverts energy from other areas. Furthermore, the anaesthetic, the medicines and the psychological trauma all take a long while to work out of the body.

The scar will remain red for two to three months, but if there is any increasing redness or pain around the wound this could indicate infection and you should contact your general practitioner or your surgeon. Work at the exercises to your arm and shoulder. If you notice any swelling of your arm on the side of the operation make sure you sleep with it raised up on a pillow, and if it has not gone down by the morning try to keep it up during the day. If it is still not normal by the following morning let your general practitioner or surgeon know.

RADIOTHERAPY

Malignant cells are more easily killed by radiation than normal cells are. If the dose of radiation is carefully adjusted, breast cancer cells that have spread to other areas of the body can usually be cleared from those areas with only mild effects on the rest of the tissues. The radiation comes as an invisible beam from a large machine containing a powerful radiation source, and this machine rotates to bombard the malignant cells from different angles, thereby reducing the effects on any individual portion of overlying skin. Another much less common way of giving radiotherapy is to implant radioactive iridium wires in the tissue for a few days and then remove them.

Radiotherapy is rarely given as a first line treatment to the primary tumour – that is better removed surgically – but it is most often used after surgery to kill small collections of cells that might remain, or it is used to deal with tumour metastases (secondary tumours), particularly ones in bones that are painful. Having radiotherapy does not necessarily mean that your specialist knows that you definitely do have remaining malignant cells in the body, just that there might be.

Only certain hospitals have radiotherapy units, so you may have to travel. You will be given an appointment to see the consultant radiotherapist who may want additional tests done, but who will then explain the plan of treatment. This treatment can only start when the operation site is fully healed.

The first session will be a planning one, when blue marks are put on the skin to outline the areas to be treated. The calculations are always different for each individual patient but it is likely you will have to attend each weekday (no treatment at weekends) for between three and five weeks.

The person who actually administers the treatment, according to the carefully calculated plan, is called a radiographer. You attend as an outpatient and each treatment session only lasts a few minutes, although inevitably there will be waiting and administration time to add to this. Once you are in position in the treatment room, everyone leaves and you are alone with the large machine, although with a microphone to talk to those outside.

The treatment, which is completely painless, often produces a delayed reaction in the skin rather like sunburn, with darkening and tenderness of the skin; to minimise this there is a ban on washing or putting creams or powders on the area being treated. This can make it become itchy, especially in hot weather. Occasionally the treatment has to be interrupted to let this reaction settle. The effects it produces on the skin usually settle completely, although the breast after radiotherapy may always be a little firmer than before.

Sometimes loss of appetite, fatigue and depression occur during treatment, usually from the strain of attending each day for so many weeks rather than the physical effects of treatment. The mental strain of radiotherapy should not be underestimated, since walking into what is very much a 'cancer clinic' and looking at the other 'cancer patients', some of whom may look very ill, takes a toll on even the strongest as the weeks go by.

So radiotherapy for breast cancer is painless and effective. It does not cause hair on your head to fall out or make you vomit, as people often suppose. We all worry about radiation, and yet here you are being exposed to very high levels. This is made possible because the radiation beam is carefully directed just to the parts of the body to be treated and has no effect on areas where it would cause damage, such as the intestine. It is also worrying when we hear that radiation can result in cancers forming, and yet here radiation is being used to cure cancer. It is true that new cancers have been produced by radiotherapy, but only very rarely and they usually arise about 20 years after treatment; on balance this is a very small risk, to be set against the chance of having your present cancer cells killed.

CHEMOTHERAPY

The word 'chemotherapy' often carries about as much dread as the word 'cancer' – we immediately think of patients with their hair falling out and vomiting. Chemotherapy actually means 'therapy by medicines', although the term is generally applied just to cancer treatments. And some of these modern medicines have almost no side effects. There are two types of chemotherapy, hormonal therapy and cytotoxic therapy.

Hormonal therapy
The commonest medicine now used against breast cancer is called tamoxifen. It was originally thought to block the stimulating effect of oestrogen on breast cancer cells, but now it seems it also blocks other cancer growth factors as well. It is certainly effective in reducing the chance of getting a recurrence. In one study of patients over 50 years who were given tamoxifen for two years, there was a 6 per cent reduction in their chance of dying of recurrent disease. It has been more difficult to show the same improvements in survival in younger women, but certainly the chance of getting a recurrence is delayed and is probably reduced overall.

The side effects of tamoxifen are so few that only 1 per cent of patients have to stop taking it and that is usually because of a little nausea. So now the majority of women are given tamoxifen, usually as an addition to their other treatments, and present recommendations are that this should be continued for two years, although more trials are needed to see if there is an advantage in continuing for even longer. Tamoxifen should not be given in pregnancy, and it does stop menstruation. However, some elderly women, whose cancers are very slow growing, are treated with tamoxifen and no operation, and this will often stop them getting any more problems from the tumour.

Before tamoxifen was available, breast cancers, and particularly recurrent ones, were treated by changing the hormone levels circulating in the blood. Oestrogen tablets were used for elderly women, while premenopausal patients were treated by removing the source of oestrogen by surgically removing the ovaries or stopping them working by radiotherapy (tamoxifen usually now makes this unnecessary). A second line of attack was to remove the adrenal glands which produce other hormones; this is also no longer necessary because of a new drug called aminoglutethimide which can be used if tamoxifen fails to control a breast cancer.

Cytotoxic drugs

The other principal type of chemotherapy uses cytotoxic drugs. These drugs kill cells but, like radiotherapy, rely for their effect on the fact that cancer cells are more susceptible than normal cells. Adjuvant chemotherapy is when these cytotoxic drugs are given at the same time as surgical treatment, in an attempt to kill any microscopic cancer deposits that might have got into the body before the tumour was removed. A combination of three drugs is usually given and there is clear evidence that if they are given for six months then the chance of dying from that cancer will be significantly reduced if looked at over a five-year period.

So why is such treatment not always given? First, it is not so effective for all women; those over 50 seem to have less benefit. Second, the side effects are troublesome, with hair loss, vomiting, nausea, bowel upsets, numb fingers, mouth ulcers, abdominal pains, malaise and vulnerability to infections. And the cost of chemotherapy also has to be taken into account. Even paying only prescription charges for the drugs you take home can come to quite a lot, and it may be cheaper for you to get a 'season ticket' for these prescriptions.

Occasionally these cytotoxic drugs are given to treat recurrent disease, but this is much rarer now that tamoxifen and aminoglutethimide are available. Also, various newer drugs are being studied and there is every reason to suppose that over the next few years trials will show some significant advances.

CLINICAL TRIALS

Many of the recent improvements in treatment – for example, cure rates obtained by lumpectomy are now as good as those obtained by radical mastectomy, and tamoxifen can further increase the number of cures – have been confirmed by clinical trials. In such trials an accepted, but new, treatment is usually tried out on a group of patients and the results compared with those for patients treated with a more familiar course of treatment. Much still needs to be worked out, though, and large numbers of people will need to be entered into trials to help develop and refine the next set of advances. For this reason most trials are now multi-centre, and sometimes international, with many hospitals collaborating. There is therefore a fair chance that you will be asked to help in such trials. It is of course difficult at a worrying time to have a doctor asking you if you will agree to help with a clinical trial; agreement to this sort of request is always entirely voluntary, however, and you will never be entered into a trial without your knowledge or consent.

Any clinical trial you are likely to be involved in will probably be comparing two well-accepted treatments, with patients being allocated at random to one or the other. For instance it might be to answer the question 'Does it offer any additional benefit if we give tamoxifen after local excision plus radiotherapy for a tumour?' One group will therefore have the well-accepted treatment of lumpectomy plus radiotherapy, together with placebo tablets (tablets that don't do anything), and the other group will have the same treatment plus tamoxifen tablets.

You can be sure that if it ever becomes clear during the course of a trial that one treatment gives significantly better results than the other, that trial would be stopped – no patient is given one treatment if it is known that another is better. All such trials are scrutinised by an ethical committee that will include lay members as well as doctors.

So find out exactly what is involved and what are the treatments being tested. If you are certain you want one of those treatments and not the other, then say so and that is what you will have. But remember, the trial would not have been started if it was known which one was best. Find out also if the clinical trial will mean additional tests or visits, or if there will be further choices of treatment later. And even if you do enter a trial, there is nothing to stop you leaving it later if you wish. In fact, the chances are that you will get even more thoroughly checked and supervised if you are in a trial than you would do otherwise, so although you will be doing this largely to help others you will probably be helping yourself as well.

PROBLEMS OVER TREATMENT

Problems and misunderstandings over treatment are rare, and you can help to prevent them by making sure you understand what is planned, what the treatment is to be and when it is intended to take place. Always ask if there is something you want to know. If you are not an inpatient in hospital you can always phone or write to your consultant to clarify a problem. If you feel you cannot accept the treatment that is planned for you, tell your specialist. It may be that there are details about your tumour you had not been aware of that affect the decision; alternatively, he may agree to follow the treatment you want.

Talking to someone who has been along this same path before is often a great help, and a volunteer visitor can be contacted through the Mastectomy Association and other agencies. However, be careful of friends telling you what they recommend; your specialist is in possession of more detailed facts than they are.

Suppose your specialist will not answer your questions, is unsympathetic or has told you something that you believe is wrong. Perhaps you think he is incompetent or perhaps he seems too certain of what he is doing for you to trust him. What do you do then? The first thing to do is to contact him directly, in person, by phone or by letter, explain the problem, and see what happens. The chances are the problem will be solved. If it is not, or if you just feel he is unsympathetic and your treatment is being affected by this, then you have every right to seek a second opinion.

Requesting a second opinion is rarely done in the UK. It can be provided free on the NHS but the problem is, first, do you have the nerve to ask, and, second, how do you go about it? If you are an outpatient then it is relatively easy – your GP can refer you to someone else. You may just want to get confirmation that the first treatment was best, in which case you can still go back to the first specialist if you wish. If you are an inpatient in a hospital it is more difficult. You will need to explain to your specialist what you want to do. Your GP may be able to recommend another specialist, or your consultant may, or perhaps you know or have had recommended someone else. It may rather sound as though you doubt the medical competence of your first specialist, but if you have explained what the problem is and it has not been resolved, then go ahead – it can often be accomplished quite simply, with no hard feelings. And doctors are often the first to accept that no two doctors will hold exactly the same opinions about how to manage a patient.

However seeking a second opinion is not a course to be taken lightly. In some countries second, third and even fourth opinions are a way of medical life, to the detriment of patient care. In such circumstances you can end up delaying treatment which should not be delayed, and causing yourself a lot of worry and uncertainty. How can you be sure that the second opinion was better than the first? Bear in mind that any problem can often be solved simply by a quiet discussion with your specialist, your GP or your nurse counsellor.

11

BREAST CANCER AFTER IT IS TREATED

COMING TO TERMS WITH WHAT HAS HAPPENED

When you first get home after treatment for breast cancer you may feel a great sense of relief and even euphoria after all the traumas you have gone through in hospital. You will probably be quietly proud of the way you took the news, and the way you coped with the operation and everything else in hospital better than you thought you would.

But so often depression and tiredness come over you when you get home. Probably for the first time you have come face to face with the fact that one day you are going to die, and that it might be much sooner than you ever supposed. That fear of death will be made even more real if you actually know someone who has died of breast cancer. If your treatment did involve a mastectomy you have the additional feelings of mourning for the loss of your breast, which has been such an important part of you, your femininity and your identity.

So thoughts of 'Why me?' keep surfacing. You will probably feel isolated. Often the lowest point comes about two months after leaving hospital, when all treatment has finished and outpatient visits have become less frequent. These feelings may continue for a long time, and sometimes anxiety and depression may become so marked that you feel there is little point, and certainly no pleasure, in going on living. This makes relationships with family and friends difficult, avoiding meeting people leads to increasing isolation, and so on, in a vicious circle. The anxiety produces insomnia, tiredness and loss of appetite, while every ache leads to worries that there might be a recurrence. Sometimes there is just anger and resentment.

103

'How can others understand? They haven't had cancer.'

However there will come a time when you can say 'I'm fine'. You will probably find that because of the way your life has been threatened, every day becomes so much more precious and you are able to live life to the full in a way you never did before. The problem is how do you get to that point?

You have to start by accepting and coming to terms with what has happened. Your thinking needs to be very positive. Don't pretend the problems are not there, or, if you have had a mastectomy, that you do not miss your breast. Do not isolate yourself – this is particularly a time when you do need others. You need people to put their arms around you and hug you, and people to involve you in fun and friendship and laughter. If you keep your sense of humour and are open and approachable, then it is easier for others to help you. If you wear attractive clothes and take trouble over your appearance people will respond, and it is wonderful for your own morale. Add to all that enough sleep and some good tiring exercise, and you will be feeling better already. Sometimes going away on a holiday helps you to put the whole episode into better perspective.

Of course all this is easier if you have made a rapid and straightforward recovery from your treatment and your wound has healed well, your arm movement is good, your prosthesis is satisfactory and you are not having continuing problems from radiotherapy or medical treatments.

TALKING TO OTHERS

The sooner you tell people what has happened, the sooner you can get help and support from them. It may be difficult to know how and when to go about it, but one consolation is that it gets easier each time you do tell someone. You will be pleased at the way some people react, bringing greater love and kindness than you could ever have imagined. Inevitably, some people will make silly thoughtless remarks, while others will seem to act awkwardly – after all, it may be as new a situation for them as it is for you. Many people will tend to take their cue from you, often waiting to see if you bring up the subject, if you want to talk, even if you want to meet people or keep to yourself. They may well stay away from you because they do not know how to react. Do not take this personally, and above all do not let yourself become isolated. Problems often arise if there are some relatives you have not confided in. When you do tell them they will be upset that they were not told sooner. Others may become overprotective when they know what has happened, and this can in itself become a great strain. There is also the problem of 'surrogate hypochondria' to deal with, when every little ache you mention, or meal you miss, raises the level of anxiety in those all around you.

A frequent source of argument arises when relatives or friends think you are not having the right treatment or seeing the right specialist. They illustrate their concern by describing the breast problems and misadventures that they or their friends have had (often the last thing you want to hear at this time). Reminding yourself that they are just trying to help is difficult, so if you find what they are saying upsets you, then tell them so.

One of the most difficult topics to talk to others about is your fear of death. If you mention it, the chances are you will quickly be told not even to think of such things – you 'must look on the bright side'. People think that to talk about death is almost to wish it on yourself – is even evidence of a disturbed mind. You will probably find the only people you can really discuss such questions with are other women who have had breast cancer themselves.

SUPPORT GROUPS

Your doctors will do their best to answer your questions, but many women leave hospital or outpatient clinics feeling confused and dissatisfied with the discussions they have had. There may have been too little time for discussions, or you may have thought at the time that some of the questions you wanted to ask were too trivial. Certainly the clinical atmosphere of the hospital is not the ideal place for quiet discussions, particularly with the number of interruptions that often take place. Perhaps you found that a male doctor just did not have a full enough understanding of your problems, or perhaps your fears and resentment were too deep-seated at the time for you to be able to express them. Doctors' expertise varies and it may be that your doctor was very skilled at administering medical treatments but less skilled at communicating with his patients. This is where others who are specially trained can help, particularly if they have been down the same path before and have special experience of these problems.

The doctor may well take the initiative and put you in touch with a volunteer helper who has had breast cancer. She may have been a patient in that particular hospital or perhaps was contacted through an organisation such as the Mastectomy Association. She will be able to give more practical help than the professional staff can, and you may find it much easier to talk to her. Some hospitals are able to provide counselling by a specially trained nurse or social worker. Sometimes these counsellors are present right at the start, when the cancer is first discovered; they provide a shoulder to cry on, they have a lot of useful information and they will discuss your fears and feelings, as well as giving you information about the support groups that you can contact when you leave hospital.

Self-help groups are able to contribute in two main ways. First, they can provide advice and practical help, such as providing you with a companion for hospital outpatient appointments, helping with transport, shopping, or looking after your children. They can also advise on the various psychological ways people have found to fight the disease itself.

Second, they can provide a forum in which you can share your feelings and find out how others have coped in similar circumstances. It is reassuring to talk to those who have gone through the same physical traumas, and who have the same feelings of fear, confusion and anger as you. The groups may be run by professionals, or by patients themselves or their relatives, who often find that helping others is a good way to help themselves, and to say 'Thank you' for all the assistance they have received.

These groups do not suit everyone, but do contact them if you think they might help you, or even if you just want to find out more information about them.

CHILDREN

It is best to be honest and open with your children, and not only explain what has happened but maybe even show them

106

the operation site. Showing emotion in front of them will do no harm. There is a natural tendency to want to protect their feelings and to hide the truth from them, but so often children's fantasies are worse than the reality. They may be worrying that you are going to die; often children think that they are the cause of any problems their parents have and that they may be blamed for them. They need time to talk about what has happened and to ask questions. Remember that words like 'cancer' and even 'death' are fairly meaningless to young children. One problem with such openness, however, is that your children may show the same frankness to people outside the family, and pass on everything you have told them about your cancer to neighbours, school friends and anyone else they meet.

The stress may affect older children in different ways. If it produces 'difficult' behaviour, try and remember that it may just be a sign of their anxiety about you. They may also be wondering about your appearance and whether it will be obvious to others that you have had a breast operation. An older daughter may be wondering about her own risk of getting breast cancer, but she may be frightened to ask. (Indeed, she will be at a slightly greater risk of getting a breast cancer.)

RELATIONSHIPS WITH MEN

If you are married you will naturally look to your husband at this difficult time for all the help and support he can give. This will be difficult because he will be going through the same emotional turmoil as you. The diagnosis will have shocked and frightened him, he will be afraid you are going to die and there will be many questions about the cancer he wants to ask but perhaps is too worried to ask or has just not had the opportunity. He may feel guilty about wanting his questions answered when you are the one with the cancer. So you need to sit down together to talk, or better still go away, perhaps for a weekend together, and talk.

If you have had a mastectomy you may be worrying that he will no longer find you physically attractive. You may worry particularly about what his reaction will be when he first sees the operation site, and how soon it is best to let him see it. If you still have any dressings when you leave the hospital it is

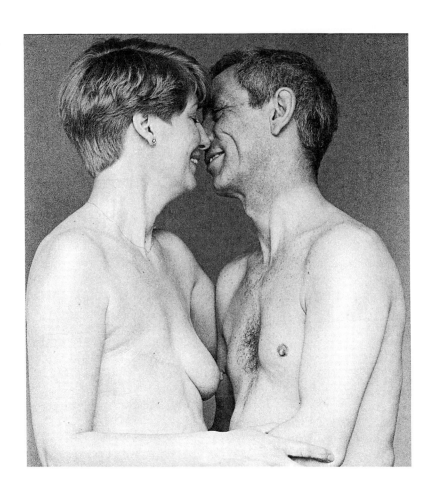

usually a good idea to ask him to help with these; that allows both of you to get used to dealing with the operation site in a matter-of-fact way. In practice it is far more likely to be anxiety about each other's reactions to the operation that comes between you than any loss of attractiveness because of the operation.

If you do not have a constant partner, then you have the advantage of not having to cope with a partner's reaction to the stress as well as your own. And any close relationship you make in the future will start with the operation being past history; you will be accepted as you are, with what has happened being just background detail. Of course you will worry that that knowledge will stop you making any such close relationships, until you realise that 'past medical history' comes near the bottom of any list of factors that affect whether someone is attracted to you or not. Any new partner will never have known your body to be any different. And if your past medical experiences do upset him, then perhaps he is not the right person for you anyway.

PHYSICAL PROBLEMS

Usually the physical problems that arise from the various treatments are easier for doctors to deal with than the psychological problems. Scars usually heal quickly these days, and wound infections are extremely rare. Often there will be some thickening of the tissues underlying a scar, and it is very easy to start wondering if this means that the lump was not properly removed. However this is a usual occurrence after a breast operation, and is just evidence of a healthy healing response. These days most scars are placed so that they are not conspicuous, even in lowcut clothes, and they should go soft and flat over about a two-month period.

Stiffness of the shoulder may occur if the scar extends to the armpit (axilla), and particularly if the lymph nodes in the armpit were removed. If a shoulder is not exercised regularly it has a natural tendency to get stiff, and in the early days after the operation you may be asked not to move it more than a certain extent. Later you may find exercise pulls on the wound and makes it ache, so by the time it is really possible to exercise fully you have a lot of work to do to regain a full range of movement. Physiotherapists in the hospital can provide a lot of help by showing you what exercises to do, and you should aim at being able to brush the back of your head. If you can't eventually manage this, or if you are not making steady progress at home, ask to visit the outpatient physiotherapy department. Exercises need to include the forearm and hand muscles as well as the shoulder. Even the muscles of the chest wall and back need working on because there is a natural tendency to stoop after such operations and this needs exercise to correct it. It is almost always possible to get the shoulder supple and strong enough to be able to play tennis and squash again if you want to.

Pains in the chest wall and arm may occur, particularly if the breast has been removed and if the armpit (axilla) has been cleared. Sometimes this is thought to be a 'phantom' pain occurring because the body has not realised that the breast is not there, but often it is because a nerve in the armpit is caught up in scar tissue. The pain may extend to the upper arm and sometimes there is an area of numbness there. It is easy to start wondering if this means that there has been spread of the cancer, but it is in fact a common postoperative problem and gradually fades with time.

Lymphoedema is swelling due to lymph accumulating in the arm because the flow of lymph is obstructed in the armpit where nodes have been removed. It makes the arm feel heavy, awkward and clumsy. In time the body will make new lymph channels and let it all drain away, providing it has not been allowed to settle in the tissues too long. If this fluid stays in the tissues for a few days the protein in the lymph stimulates fibrosis in the arm, and the swelling can become permanent. What you must do is be sure that it drains away each night by making use of gravity. So at night raise the arm on a pillow, or even arrange for it to be held up by a towel wrapped round it, so that the lymph can flow downhill to the shoulder. If the swelling has not all gone by the morning you must rest with it up during the day or see your doctor for an elastic sleeve to compress the arm.

Another problem with this swelling is that it encourages infection, which in turn generates more swelling. So take the greatest care of the arm, being especially careful when cutting your nails, and putting antiseptic cream on any little cuts. At the first sign of redness visit your doctor, because you may need antibiotics.

PROSTHESES

If your operation has involved a mastectomy, you can get a breast prosthesis to fit into your bra. It should feel soft and comfortable, and when you are dressed it should be impossible for anyone to tell that you have had a breast operation. There are about 14 different types of breast prosthesis and the best ones are gel filled. They are able to match the other breast very closely in shape, weight and consistency, they change

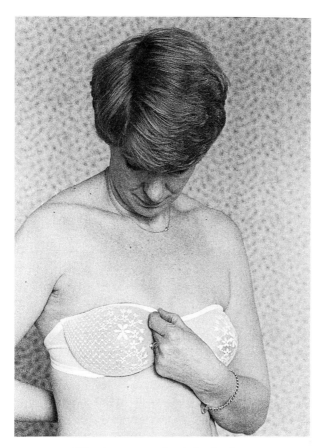

Wearing a prosthesis in the bra.

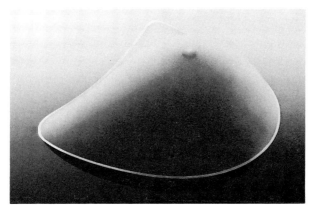

Gel-filled prosthesis.

shape as you move, and are not cold but take on the same temperature as the rest of the body.

Surgeons are often not very knowledgeable about the different types of prosthesis, and fitting you with one is often left to the appliance officer. If the one you get is not comfortable or satisfactory then go back to the appliance officer – prostheses are provided by the NHS in any type or size needed and may be replaced as often as necessary. It should also be possible for you to go swimming with a prosthesis, preferably sewn into your custume so that you can feel completely safe that it will not slip.

It is difficult even to get measured up for a prosthesis when the scar is still tender, so the definitive prosthesis is usually left for a fortnight or so after the operation. In the meantime a soft temporary one is used.

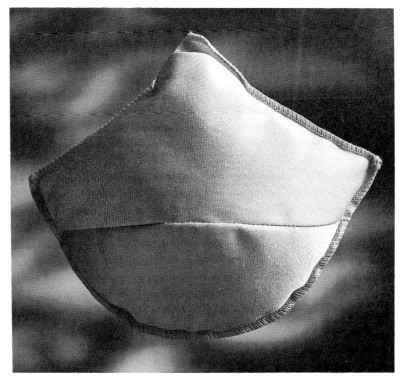

Soft temporary prosthesis for wearing immediately after the operation.

Seeing a prosthesis for the first time will probably remind you of what you have lost and what a poor substitute an artificial breast is. There is also something rather unpleasant about the emphasis on looking normal on the outside, as though the only importance of breasts is that they should look all right to others and that nothing else matters. There are some women who do not wear a prosthesis because they do not wish to hide away their loss. Here again talking to others who have been through this before can help you to decide for yourself what you want to do.

FOLLOW-UP VISITS

After the treatment is over you will naturally be visiting your general practitioner. Although he will have had reports from the hospital, he will wish to hear from you what has happened and how you are progressing. There may be medicines you need to get from him, and certificates for work, and there may be some questions you want to ask that you did not get clear answers to in hospital. The closer he is kept in touch with all your progress the more he can help.

You will also be given an outpatient appointment for the hospital. The usual arrangement is for you to be seen at three-month intervals on two or three occasions and then six-monthly intervals, until finally the intervals may be nine or twelve months, although this varies considerably for different patients. You may have appointments to attend two different clinics, perhaps surgical and radiotherapy. As well as being asked about any new symptoms and having a physical examination at each visit, there may be blood tests and X-rays.

Often you will have put the operation behind you and then one of these appointments comes along and reminds you all about it again. Going back to the same hospital and seeing the specialist again brings back all the anxieties about the disease. It reminds you that the tumour might recur. Often it means a wait in a crowded clinic and then an apparently rather cursory examination, perhaps by a new member of the team that you have not met before. You may even receive slightly different advice, that conflicts with advice you received on earlier visits.

Of course looking for a recurrence of the cancer is by no means the only reason for these outpatient visits. Early on

113

there may be problems with the scar, stiffness of the shoulder or problems with the arm to sort out. Medicines may need their doses altered, or they may need to be changed. There may be difficulties with the prosthesis that need sorting out, and you may want to discuss the question of breast reconstruction. It is a time when you can ask questions you forgot to ask before.

Of course, there will be checks to make sure that cancer has not returned. It is important to find a local recurrence in the operation site early, especially if it has been a lumpectomy operation. Screening checks on the other breast will be done to make sure there is no new cancer there, probably with mammograms every two years. It might seem as though it would be the last straw to develop a second breast cancer, but remember that it will be just as curable as the first, and the cure could be with even greater certainty if you find the cancer early. You will therefore be shown how you can check the operation site yourself and how to examine the other breast.

Do not delay reporting new symptoms merely because you know you are under outpatient review. If you do find something, do not wait until the next appointment before reporting it – that may be months away. Report any new symptoms immediately; probably go to your GP first, and he or she will know what is important.

So there are good reasons for these follow-up visits. Think of them just as a routine part of the treatment, and not that you are a special case at special risk. If it is found, at regular intervals, that all is well then at least this is worth hearing. And finally, of course, it is helpful for the specialists to know how successful their treatments are by reviewing their patients.

RECURRENCE

The majority of recurrences of breast cancer occur in the first year or two after diagnosis and treatment, but there is never a time when you can say for certain that you are beyond the stage when the cancer might recur. Even though the chances of a recurrence get smaller and smaller as time goes on, it is still possible to get a recurrence 20 or more years after the operation. This is because the body's defences have been able to keep a check on the few remaining cancer cells – have kept them under control and lying dormant – until for some reason

114

they become unable to do this any longer. This is why so much importance is attached to tamoxifen and adjuvant chemotherapy (see page 99) and to generally keeping fit and healthy, in an attempt to reduce the chance of this happening. The chance of a recurrence varies for each individual, depending on the size of the original tumour, whether lymph nodes were involved, etc.

In fact, it is not even particularly important to an individual whether they have an x per cent chance of a recurrence; what matters most is what actually happens to them. Moreover, the figures we have now for recurrence rates 10 or 20 years after an operation relate to treatments carried out before many of the recent developments were introduced. It is therefore reasonable to suppose that there will be some improvement when today's figures finally get analysed.

How a recurrence would show itself depends on where it occurs. It might produce a change that you notice, such as a pain or a lump, possibly a cough or shortness of breath, or maybe just loss of appetite or a drop in weight. The lump might be in the region of the operation or in the associated lymph nodes. Sometimes the recurrence is found in a completely different part of the body; this is because a few cancer cells escaped from the tumour before it was removed and were transported around the body in the blood or lymph channels. Sometimes a recurrence is only found by examination or special tests at the outpatient follow-up appointments.

A natural reaction when you find that a recurrence of the cancer has been discovered is to feel very angry that after going through all the surgery and other time-consuming treatments, the tumour has come back. You may also feel scared that this time perhaps the cancer will win. Sometimes a recurrence at the operation site can be excised with hardly any greater chance of further problems. However with larger recurrences it is not usually possible to get a cure; the aim here is to get the tumour into a state of remission, whereby it remains dormant for years. Today's treatments can often produce remissions of many years, by the use of drugs such as tamoxifen, other chemotherapy agents (either cytotoxics or drugs such as aminoglutethimide that alter the blood steroids) and sometimes with the addition of radiotherapy.

115

ALTERNATIVE MEDICINE

The aim of the alternative cancer treatments is to recruit and perhaps boost the body's defences to help kill cancer cells wherever they may be in the body. Of course cancer cells are being killed all the time by the body's defences, but whether this can be increased by someone 'taking control' over their body is not yet proved. Those who teach alternative medicine aim to do this firstly by making you think and act more positively. Often patients feel that they are expected to be too passive in conventional medicine, just to hand over responsibility for their body to the professionals and let them get on with it. A study reported in the *Lancet* in 1985 showed a better 10-year survival rate if there was more determination and 'fighting spirit' and less a feeling of hopelessness – mental attitude was the most significant individual factor in prognosis (the prediction of the course of the disease). Also a study of 283 women with breast cancer showed that those with more social involvement and who coped better with problems and maintained good relationships tended to live longer. This does not prove that mental attitude killed cancer cells, but it certainly suggests that a positive attitude is a good thing.

Another common feature of the alternative medicine approach is change of diet. Although there is evidence that the development of breast cancer is related to increased intake of animal fat, there is no reason to suppose that cutting out animal fats will affect the course of the disease once it has started. Many of the suggested diets are vegetarian. Eating a healthy diet and maintaining strength and general body fitness are certainly important means of improving the body's defences, but one trouble with some of the suggested diets is that they have such low levels of protein and calories that they can actually weaken you. Also major changes of diet can be very isolating at the meal table, and can make going out to visit family or friends difficult. Visiting these different groups and buying their diets and dietary supplements can be expensive. It is a field in which quacks can make easy money and you need to be on your guard.

It is always sad for medical staff to see people giving up the treatment that has been prescribed and trying unproven therapies instead. Most doctors have come across patients who claim to have been 'cured' of cancer, but on investigation the original diagnosis of cancer had often never been proved. Spontaneous cure is extremely rare, but a remission, when a cancer stops growing for a certain period and perhaps shrinks, is not uncommon, and occurs particularly with breast cancer. The remission may last for many years.

So take what you want from these different treatments and find what suits you. Thinking positively, eating sensibly and avoiding stress are all important measures to take, but they ought to be thought of as complementary rather than alternative.

12

BREAST DISEASE IN MEN

Breast problems in men are rare, but there are two main types, benign breast enlargement, known as gynaecomastia, and cancer.

GYNAECOMASTIA

Enlargement of the male breast causes considerable embarrassment. It is not uncommon in newborn babies, and may be associated with a small amount of nipple discharge called 'witch's milk'; this is a common occurrence and clears on its own. Also, at puberty a small breast nodule may appear, which usually disappears within 18 months.

Gynaecomastia in adults may be caused by many factors but in the majority of men who develop it there is no obvious cause or hormonal disturbance. Something has just stimulated the tiny remnant of breast tissue under the nipple to grow and it is always difficult to predict how large it will become.

Sometimes, however, a cause can be found. Excessive consumption of alcohol can lead to gynaecomastia, as can many other conditions that damage the liver. A variety of medicines can cause it too; for example, apart from the obvious sex hormones, the commonest drugs causing this are spironolactone, used in heart conditions, cimetidine, used to treat stomach ulcers, various other heart drugs, and some antidepressants. Marijuana and heroin can also stimulate the growth of breast tissue in men, and it may be a feature of obesity.

It also occurs in conditions where the testes are underdeveloped, not functioning properly, or damaged by trauma or disease. In these conditions there is a shortage of the male hormone, testosterone, or an excess of the female hormone, oestrogen. Another very rare cause is a condition called Klinefelter's syndrome, which results from the presence of one or more extra X chromosomes in a man. (Chromosomes are the strands of inherited genetic material found in each cell.) The X chromosomes are the female ones, and Y chromosomes are the male ones. Normal men have one X and one Y chromosome in each cell, while women have two X chromosomes. There are a variety of ways in which the sex chromosomes can be wrongly arranged, and in Klinefelter's syndrome the pattern is usually XXY or XXXY. The result is a man with small infertile genital organs, mental retardation, and often gynaecomastia. Men with this condition also have an increased frequency of breast cancer. Finally, a very rare cause of gynaecomastia is a testicular tumour that is producing oestrogen.

Any man who has breast enlargement should be investigated – he should be asked about any drug-taking, his blood should be tested to see how the liver is functioning, and his hormone levels measured. The possibility of cancer should also be considered, although in practice this does not occur under the age of 30 in men. If there is a definite cause for the breast enlargement it should obviously be treated; however, in many cases nothing is found, and so treatment is then aimed at relieving embarrassment. The cosmetic results of surgery in men are usually good; the incision is normally made around the edge of the areola, and the breast tissue removed through it. The scar is small, and usually almost invisible.

BREAST CANCER IN MEN

Breast cancer in men is very rare. In the UK there are about 120 cases a year, compared with 29,000 in women. The causes in men are less well understood than those of women; because it is so rare, it is virtually impossible to conduct any meaningful research into it. It is likely that it is caused by changes in hormone levels, but this has been difficult to prove. Certainly, the fact that it responds well to removal of the testes (orchidectomy) suggests that hormones are involved. It has also been suggested that men who receive hormone treatment for cancer of the prostate are at an increased risk. Gynaecomastia itself has been suggested as a risk factor for breast cancer, but without convincing evidence. It is not known whether a family history is important as studies so far show conflicting results – some giving a positive association and others none at all.

Men develop cancer of the breast at a later age than women, on average by 10 years, it being most common between 60 and 70. It is usually found to be a small lump in the region of the areola, sometimes with a nipple discharge. However, it tends to be more aggressive in men, with poorer survival rates than in women.

Breast cancer in men is sometimes treated by surgery, to remove the tumour and often the underlying muscle and the lymph nodes. Radiotherapy is not particularly successful, but surgical removal of the testes does prolong survival in up to 60 per cent of cases. In addition, early trials have shown that tamoxifen appears to be effective.

FURTHER READING

Breast Cancer: The Facts, Michael Baum
Oxford University Press, 1981
A book about all aspects of breast cancer, by one of the
United Kingdom's leading breast specialists.

Breast Cancer Screening – report to the health ministers of
England, Wales, Scotland and Northern Ireland by a
working group chaired by Professor Sir Patrick Forrest
HMSO, 1986
This report has been the basis of the proposed breast-cancer
screening programme in the United Kingdom.

Breast Cancer: A Woman's Handbook, Deborah Dewar
And Books, Indiana, 1983
Written by a woman who has had breast cancer; it also
describes other women's experiences. Informative and
practical approach.

Breast Is Best, Drs Penny and Andrew Stanway
Pan, 1983
A comprehensive look at all aspects of breastfeeding, with
much practical advice.

Contraception: Your Questions Answered, John Guillebaud
Pitman, 1985
A somewhat more technical look at all aspects of
contraception.

The Pill, John Guillebaud
Oxford University Press, 1984
The combined and progestogen only pills explained in detail but in terms anyone can understand.

Successful Breastfeeding, Joan Neilson
Sheldon Press, 1985
A short simple guide to breastfeeding, concentrating on the practical aspects.

Women and Cancer, edited by Steven D. Stellman
Harrington Park Press, 1987
A series of articles dealing with aspects of several cancers. Breast self-examination, mastectomy and epidemiology of breast cancer are discussed.

USEFUL ADDRESSES AND ORGANISATIONS

Association of Breastfeeding Mothers
131 Mayow Road
Sydenham
London SE26 4HZ
Provides counselling and information service for the general
public and health professionals. Please send stamped
addressed envelope.

The Breast Care and Mastectomy Association
26 Harrison Street
King's Cross
London WC1H 8JG
01-837 0908
Provides an information and counselling service for women
who have had, or are being advised to have, a mastectomy.
Advice on clothes and prostheses is given, and a selection
can be seen on the premises. Also provide volunteers who
will visit to offer practical advice and support.

British Association of Cancer United Patients (BACUP)
121–3 Charterhouse Street
London EC1M 6AA
01-608 1661/1785
Provides information and advice about cancer.

Cancer Aftercare and Rehabilitation Society (CARE)
Lodge Cottage
Church Lane
Timsbury
Bath BA3 1LF
0761 70731
An organisation staffed by people who have had cancer.
Offers information and support.

Cancer Help Centre
Cornwallis Grove
Grove House
Clifton
Bristol BS8 4PG
0272 743216

Cancer Link
46A Pentonville Road
London N1 9HF
01-833 2451
Provides information about cancer, and also self-help and
support groups.

Family Planning Association and **Family Planning
Information Service**
27–35 Mortimer Street
London W1N 7RJ
01-636 7866
Information and leaflets on all aspects of family planning,
and other aspects of women's health.

Health Education Authority
Hamilton House
Mabledon Place
London WC1H 9TX
01-631 0930
Free leaflets on self-examination and cancer.

La Leche League of Great Britain
PO Box BM 3424
London WC1V 6XX
01-404 5011
Information, advice and leaflets on breastfeeding. Also
supplies breast pumps.

The London Centre for Psychotherapy
19 Fitzjohns Avenue
London NW3 5JY
01-435 0873
A registered charity providing individual or group
psychotherapy and counselling, at moderate fees. They take
self-referrals as well as referrals from doctors.

Margaret Pyke Centre for Study and Training in Family Planning
15 Bateman's Buildings
Soho Square
London W1V 5TW
01-734 9351
The largest centre in Europe, dealing with all aspects of family planning counselling and screening.

Marie Curie Memorial Foundation
28 Belgrave Square
London SW1 8QG
01-235 3325
Provides a nationwide domiciliary service and nursing homes for cancer patients. Also information and leaflets.

The National Childbirth Trust
9 Queensborough Terrace
London W2 3TB
01-221 3833
Information, advice and leaflets on breastfeeding. Also sells a nursing bra and supplies breast pumps.

National Society for Cancer Relief
15-19 Britten Street
London SW3 3TY
01-351 7811
Provides financial assistance for patients and relatives in need through its Patient Grant Department. Applications should be made by local authority, hospital or hospice social workers. The society also funds home care (Macmillan) nurses in the community and in National Health Service hospitals.

The Patients' Association
Room 33
18 Charing Cross Road
London WC2
01-240 0671

Relate (formerly National Marriage Guidance Council)
Head Office
Herbert Gray College
Little Church Street
Rugby
Warwicks CV21 3AP
0788 73241
Local branches can be found in telephone directories.
Provides a confidential counselling service for people who
have difficulties or anxieties in their marriage or in other
personal relationships.

Scottish Health Education Group
Woodburn House
Canaan Lane
Edinburgh EH10 4SG
031-447 8044
Similar to Health Education Authority.

Scottish Marriage Guidance Council
26 Frederick Street
Edinburgh EH2 2JR
031-225 5006
Similar to Relate formerly the National Marriage Guidance
Council, with local branches.

Women's Health Concern
17 Earl's Terrace (ground floor)
London W8 6LP
01-602 6669
Information and leaflets on all aspects of women's health.

Women's Health Information Centre
52 Featherstone Street
London EC1Y 8RT
01-251 6580/6332
Information, leaflets and addresses of local organisations.

Women's National Cancer Control Campaign
1 South Audley Street
London W1Y 5DQ
01-499 7532
Information and leaflets on breast screening, self-examination, etc. Also provide videos, for example on screening.

Private screening clinics
Marie Stopes House
The Well Woman Centre
108 Whitfield St
London W1
01-388 0662/2585

Marie Stopes Centre
10 Queen Square
Leeds LS2 8AJ
0532 440685

Marie Stopes Centre
1 Police St
Manchester M2 7LQ
061-832 4250

PPP Female Health Screening
99 New Cavendish St
London W1M 7FQ
01-637 8941

BUPA Women's Unit
300 Gray's Inn Rd
London WC1X 8DU
01-837 6484

Medical Express
Chapel Place
Oxford St
London W1H 9HN
01-499 1991

EIRE

Irish Family Planning Clinic
Cathal Brugha Street Clinic
Dublin 1
Dublin 727276/727363
Provides a similar service to the FPA within the confines of
Irish law.

UNITED STATES

Planned Parenthood Federation of America (head office)
2010 Massachusetts Avenue
NW Suite 500
Washington DC 20036
202 785 3351

Western region:
333 Broadway
3rd Floor
San Francisco
California 94133
415 956 8856

Northern region:
2625 Butterfield Rd
Oak Brook
Illinois 60521
312 986 9270

Southern region:
3030 Peachtree Road
NW Room 303
Atlanta
Georgia 30305

AUSTRALIA

Australian Federation of FPAs
Suite 603
6th Floor
Roden Cutler House
24 Campbell St
Sydney
NSW 2000

NEW ZEALAND

The New Zealand FPA Inc.
PO Box 68200
214 Karangahape
Newton
Auckland

SOUTH AFRICA

FPA of South Africa
412 York House
46 Kerk St
Johannesburg 2001

INDEX

Numbers in *italics* refer to illustrations.

133

pectoralis major, 66
pectoralis muscle, 1, *2*, 88
pelvis, 90
periods, 9
pethedine, 46, 55
physical problems, 109
physical trauma, 106
physiotherapists, 95, 109
pigmentation, 42
pituitary gland, 4, 6
placebo tablets, 100
plastic surgeon, 33, 65
plastic surgery: x, 71; prior
    considerations, 65
poisons, 84
poorly differentiated, 82
'popping', 66, 70
positive thinking, 104, 116
powders, 97
pregnancy, 4, 6, 29, 42–3, 62, 74, 99
pregnancy, late age, 60
premature babies, 55
premenstrual heaviness, ix
premenstrual tenderness, 19
premenstrual tension, 20
primary tumour, 84, 90
problems and treatment, 101–2
progesterone, 6
progestogen, 20, 22, 49, 58, 61, 62
progestogen-only pill (POP), 58, 62
prognosis, 116
prolactin, 6, 20, 22, 46
prostate, 120
prostheses, 65, 110–13, *111*
prosthesis, 66, 69, 81, 95, 104
prosthesis, temporary, *112*
protein, 116
proteins, 56
protractile nipples, 53
pseudoephedrine, 49
psychological trauma, 96
puberty, 4–5, 118
puffiness, 10, 14, 34

radiation, 17, 76, 80, 96
radioactive iridium wires, 96
radiographer, 40, 97
radiotherapist, 86, 90
radiotherapy, 83, 88, 89, 96–8, 99,
    104, 113, 115, 120
recurrence, 114
relationships, 103, 107, 116
remission, 115, 117
resentment, 103, 105
retroviruses, 79
ribs, 1, *2*, 29, 35

sagging, 62
sarcoma, 72
saturated fats, 21
scars, 31, 67, 109, 114
scirrhous, 82
screening, 7, 39, 81, 114
screening clinics, 14
sebaceous glands, 2, 42
secondary tumours, 84, 85, 89, 97
secretion, 2
sedatives, 49
self-esteem, 64
self-examination, 7–8, *9*, 10, *10*, 11,
    11, 80
self-help groups, 106
serum, 79
sexual arousal, 3, 5
sexual role, 57
shape of breast, 1
shingles, 29, 34
shoulder, 109, 114
side-effects of drugs, 21, 22
silicone gel implants, 65, 69
silicone prosthesis, 70
skin, 33, 36, 54, 97
smoking, 50
social class, 76
specialist, 90, 102
spine, 29, 90
spironolactone, 118
staphylococci, 25
statistics, 60, *73*, 75
steriods, 115
stress, 77
stretch marks, 4
stretching, 42
structure of breast, 1
suckling, 47, *48*, 49, 55
support groups, 105
surgeons, 91, 96
surgery, 37, 69, 89
surgical breast augmentation, 5
surgical breast reduction, 5
surgical correction, 33
'surrogate hypochondria', 105
suspensory ligaments, 14, 15, 31, 68
swelling, 58, 110
symptoms, 114

talking, 104
tamofixen, 21, 81, 83, 88, 98, 99, 100,
    115, 120
tenderness, ix, 5, 6, 19, 20, 23, 29, 30,
    33, 36, 58, 59
testes, 118, 119
testosterone, 119

134